How to Live Happily Ever After "Down Under"

How to Live Happily Ever After "Down Under"

The How To Thrive With Lichen Sclerosis Guide

Tammie Quick

ISBN: 0995080100
ISBN 13: 9780995080102

Acknowledgements

WHEN I WAS a little kid I could not bring myself to pick a "favourite" colour because I worried that all of the other colours would feel left out. This acknowledgement business is no different! My goodness… how to remember everyone and know what particular order to place them in is complete madness! But here goes:

If you have loved me; challenged me; married me; parented me; shared parents with me; taught me; been born to me; fostered by me; entrusted your health care to me; or read me (Oh! And if you're a certain Tibetan Monk) – I love you and am so grateful for your participation in my journey.

And a special "shout out!" to Christiane, Cam, Ally, Sara & John for your priceless contributions to this book.

Table of Contents

Forward

Lichen Sclerosis (LS) affects women ten times more often than men. More often than not this invasive condition will show up as dry, rough, raised white spots on the individual's genitals. The eczema-like rash can be rough, red, and dotted with white raised spots like small mushroom caps.

The most debilitating part is that the itch can drive a perfectly sane gal mad. The other problem is that the lichen complex, or simplex, can be part of a greater pathology like psoriasis, erosive lichen planus, vitiligo, morphea, anemia, alopecia and even skin cancer.

In nature, when a tree has excessive lichen it is usually indicative of a deeper disease process. It is not normal, or healthy, for us to host other needy organisms that suck from our resources, especially as busy moms wives and workers with quite often several jobs, both paid and unpaid.

The allopathic community has no idea what causes LS, so a proper diagnosis of the underlying cause still remains at large in their world. Still worse, the drug treatment protocols of recommended immune modulating meds and cortisone creams will further exacerbate the issue, destroying one's immune function and thinning the already thin skin.

Both are limited conventions suppressing the root cause and inviting other outbreaks in the body. Medicines, whether allopathic or so called alternative, only have certain courses of action - suppressive, palliative or curative. Immune system modulators and cortisone are not curative.

Even the fear of not knowing can drive the sufferer's immune function into a quandary of fight or flight gestures, further exacerbating the issue. When we're in chronic pain or scratching until we bleed, we can feel utterly forsaken. When it is occurring on one's genitals it will become the deepest source of shame.

Tammie Quick does a brilliant job of taking the reader by the hand and leading them home through the portal of suffering to a sound place of regimen, natural medicine and therapeutic education. The best part is that you'll feel like you're sitting in a comfortable café chatting with your closest girlfriend about your girlie bits.

Tammie starts by telling you her own profound tale of suffering and then opens the door wide for protocols that she knows can provide you with both temporary and then permanent relief. Although, she draws those lines clearly, she also empowers her reader to pick and choose from her pharmacy of care and experience.

This book, on this debilitating affliction is so accessible - having been stripped of any false authority or medical jargon. If you suffer from LS, you will have the dynamic answers in this clear and concise read. From what the cause is, to how to treat the issue at home naturally (without causing yourself more harm), to fermented foods and supplements to heal from the inside out, to what to wash your undergarments with to prevent exacerbating your condition further.

In essence you get a highly experienced naturotherapist with years of study, and experience, combined with the feeling that you've just made a new best friend, all within these pages. I know that you'll love Tammie's approach, especially if you're *secretly* suffering LS symptoms, privately afflicted with shame and embarrassment.

It was while I was reading Tammie's own history of how she may have contracted Lichen Sclerosis by repeated rounds of antibiotics and sulpha drugs in childhood that my own wheels began turning. Like the Author, I too suffered repeated bouts of tonsillitis; kidney and bladder infections as a child back in the 1960's and 70's.

No one blinked an eye when I was put on several rounds of antibiotics or courses of Monistat for yeast infections beginning at the age of twelve. As a result, I suffered an overgrowth of vaginal yeast exacerbated by my overly tight jeans (the style at the time) - the yellow laden discharge in the gusset of my panties, a telltale sign that the underlying cause was still at large.

Oh those shame-filled moments of having to tell my step-mother that the horrible issue was back, yet again. Not being able to squelch the itch that was beyond embarrassing (and also painful), affected my confidence and later, my capacity for intimacy. And the odor of being sick in my privates affected every aspect of my natural sexual development at a critical time in my feminine unfolding.

Tammie is the first person that I've met that I've exposed this history to in writing and it was by reading her book that I stepped up, in solidarity with my fellow sufferer. When you read her story, you'll know why. She's made me feel safe, encouraged and empowered to do so. And if you're a sufferer of LS, you will perhaps want to share your story to help another fellow sufferer too. At the very least, you'll give them this book as you'll feel so excited to finally have found a knowledgeable confidant through Tammie's words.

I also know that this is how Tammie's patients feel about her as well. I know because Tammie and I studied together during a four year plus medical degree in Heilkunst Medicine. We've seen testimonials from her beloved patients, having experienced a whole variety of cures in her capable care.

If you should need a warm knowledgeable hand to guide you to a resolution with your LS suffering, I know that she can work with you both near and by far using Skype or the phone. You'd never regret it as she is very much like a modern medical Monk with abounding compassion. She is the Physician who truly has healed thyself.

For now, you will love having the opportunity to obtain this knowledge through Tammie's book. It truly will be one of the most pleasurable, even humour-filled, reads you'll ever have.

Not only will you find the answers you seek, but you will share this book with countless other sufferers who dare to come forward. You will welcome your mother, sister, daughter and friend into our burgeoning sisterhood of Lichen Sclerosis sufferers with open arms. I'm happy to be counted amongst her very brave numbers and to be healed by Tammie's knowledge-filled words.

Allyson McQuinn, DHHP, JAOH
Doctor of Medical Heilkunst and Author
(http://arcanum.ca/AMcQuinn)

Introduction

WHAT IS A miracle? I'm sure that the dictionary (or Google!) would have a different definition than mine, but here goes: A miracle is something that happens that changes your life in a – in a most unusual and unpredictable way, for the better. It is a life-altering event so dramatic and surreal that it is considered to have come from God or the universe, or some deity.

Such an event happened to me.

It was well past midnight one August night. I had gotten up because I couldn't sleep, the itching was that bad. It had been pretty bad for most of the day but often my life activities would keep my mind off of it. I had managed not to scratch for the entire day, which meant that my skin was nearly healed up again from scratching the last time. It was almost impossible not to scratch. The impulse to do so was like being horny. There's a reason that arousal has been described as "an itch you can't scratch". Or maybe it was a Lichen Sclerosis sufferer that coined that term! Learning Homeopathy meant that I'd become intimately familiar with the term "voluptuous itching" and boy did I experience that!! But unlike sex, scratching brought intense but fleeting pleasure to be replaced by much pain until the healing got to the point of intense itching again, instead of pain. What a vicious cycle! This had become my life. Scratch, pain, heal, itch, fight the itch, lose the battle; begin again.

I tried so many potions and lotions and different therapies… everything from talk therapy to Bodytalk (another form of talk therapy I guess!), to food restrictions, to supplements, and Homeopathy of course!

In many ways, I was so much better, but the itching and scratching wasn't. It never got better. It was my dirty little secret for probably close to 18 years, though at first it wasn't all the time. But certainly for about 13 years it had been a chronic, constant companion... and it was getting worse.

Back to that night, there was a spot right near my tail bone. I was walking away from the bedroom heading to the family room to distract myself with TV. Oh but that spot was calling so loudly that I couldn't think of anything else! Surely I would be fine with just a little scratching, just near the spot, not on it? But I wasn't. I only scratched through my nightgown, so that I wouldn't break the skin and I always kept my fingernails short, but soon there was a lot of blood on my nightgown. And I guess the combination of the itching (like a bad lover touching me and calling out to me relentlessly all day – one I tried to ignore; one that I didn't want to be excited by but I couldn't help it cause my body betrayed me) plus seeing the blood kind of made me lose my mind. I started scratching everything... every part that longed to be scratched and mutilated, was going to be satisfied on this hot August night. It was so bad. I was crying and feeling utterly ashamed and hopeless. I jumped into the bathtub and ran the water to calm the pain, and there was blood running down my legs. It was hurting so much but the scratching was also intensely pleasurable. It must have been an act of God that made me finally stop, because I was a crazy person who had given over to the temptation of the dark side, and I could not.

I had never hurt myself like this before. I was disgusted and worried about my partner's reaction because he would be leaving for work out of town the next day, and wanting intimacy between us before he drove off. Now I wouldn't be able to accommodate him. So many times in our 20 plus year relationship I hadn't been able to. Or when I did, we had to be extremely careful of breaking my delicate skin... or worse, of waking the monster.

If the "danger zone" of the folds between my legs and my genitals was accidentally touched, I'd go crazy and start to scratch while we were making love.

He told me that it was like being in bed with a banshee… at first a little erotic but then kind of frightening. I hated my life. My entire life revolved around Lichen Sclerosis.

After I somehow re-gained control and cleaned up, I went to my computer and typed out a hate letter to God. I really did. I cried and I screamed (silently and into the words); I threatened; I swore and I begged. Some days later God answered… in the form of a Tibetan monk who called me out of the blue, and offered to start working with me over the phone, to help me heal my blocked (first and second) chakras, and to help me become who I was meant to be.

That was the beginning of my miracle. I know it sounds crazy but that's what happened, and no I didn't have to send money anywhere or sign up for an online course or anything like that. It was and continues to be, my "miracle".

But that spiritual journey in its entirety, is a book for another day. Today I share the healing part of my spiritual journey back from the edge of Lichen Sclerosis Hell…

After my rant to God, I resigned myself to getting a prescription for some cortisone cream (so I could get some sleep!), and to see a dermatologist to be diagnosed because while I was suspicious that I suffered from Lichen Sclerosis, when I'd asked my M.D. about it years before, he didn't even know what it was.

Of course the cortisone helped but it didn't cure it. I was very nervous about using it because of my medical training and because I am a sensitive, fair-skinned, red-head (or so they tell me, but I've always preferred the term strawberry-*blonde!*) who reacts to everything. So I only used the tiniest amount and only once daily. But after several hours, that familiar twinge began to start travelling up my sensitive nerve endings again. And while the skin did heal, it never quite felt right, plus it was getting thinner… which dermatologists say is a necessary part of LS treatment because you build up so much scar tissue, but it was getting awfully easy to get wounded during intimacy or even from exercising. And after only 2 months my hair (on my head) started to fall out and I began having a full period every 2 weeks. It was clear to me that my endocrine system didn't like the synthetic cortisone very much. So I stopped it.

This guide is what I've come up with as a treatment plan, instead of cortisone cream. It may not be for everyone, and certainly you need to check with your doctor before you stop any prescribed treatment and/or medication, or before deciding to try any of the suggestions in this book.

Really, this is a sharing and it may provide information, relief and ultimately hope for LS sufferers. Please do not take it as medical advice but more as entertainment!

CHAPTER 1

What is Lichen Sclerosis (LS)?

WHAT DOES GOOGLE say:

> Lichen (noun) is defined as a skin disease in which small pimples or bumps occur close together.

> Sclerosis is a hardening or thickening of organs, tissues, or vessels from chronic inflammation, abnormal growth of fibrous tissue, or degeneration of the myelin sheath of nerve fibres.

Hmm, so a skin disease that involves thickening from chronic inflammation. Sounds about right… except they left out the itching!

Elizabeth G. Stewart M.D. and Paula Spencer describe Lichen Sclerosis (LS) in *The V Book* (Bantam books 2002)…

"The most frequent sign of vulvar LS is itching. Sometimes there is burning, and intercourse can be painful, often because of cracks in the skin near the vaginal opening.

The first change is a flat ivory-white area, irregular in shape with a little depression, in the middle. This may be on the labia, near the clitoris, on the perineum, or anywhere else on the vulva. There may be several white areas or they may blend together to form a larger area. Within the white areas, purple bruising and a thin, wrinkled appearance may be noted. (The thin, wrinkly skin is often compared to cigarette paper that people roll tobacco in.) The whitened areas may go on to thicken or thin out, sometimes to the point of creating an open sore (ulceration). In some cases the inflammation can cause the normal anatomy of the vulva to change, with flattening of the labia minora, fusion of the hood over the clitoris so that it is buried under the skin, and shrinkage of the skin around the vaginal opening. The whitening may extend down around the anus so that a white figure eight runs from the top of the labia, down their length, over the perineum, and around the anus. LS in the anal area may cause itching, cracking and bleeding of the skin, and discomfort with bowel movements. Women often think that they have hemorrhoids. Some women have even had surgery for anal cracking (fissures) or hemorrhoids when their problems came from LS the whole time! Involvement of the groin folds, thighs, and buttocks are common. It is generally accepted that LS does not involve the vagina."

I mentioned the thickening (definition of Sclerosis) not just for obvious reasons for those who suffer from LS, but because it deserves some consideration. In the Heilkunst Homeopathic system of medicine (the one that I work in) we take our patients on a journey back through time to uncover and treat the various shocks and traumas that have occurred over a lifetime. While dermatologists and other clinicians don't understand what causes LS, it is generally believed that a trauma may have preceded the development of this pathology. The trauma could be as horrific as sexual assault but it could also be as "normal" as the birth of a child, or even a routine pap test, a medication, or sex with a loving partner.

Dr. Wilhelm Reich (1897-1957) an Austrian psychoanalyst and scientist who studied under (and arguably exceeded) Freud, taught that neurosis is the consequence when human beings develop blockages throughout the body as a response to trauma and/or the need to conform to the norms of society. He called these blockages **Armoring** and said that it is the response of the organism when the normal flow of life energy has been cut off.

I am doing super-simplistic paraphrasing of a highly controversial and brilliant science. For more understanding of Wilhem Reich's work consider reading his books: The Function Of The Orgasm, The Invasion of Compulsory Sex-Morality; Character Analysis and many more. Also a simple Google search of his name will lead you to lots of learning opportunities! Do be discriminating however, as many did not understand his work and (still) seek to destroy his reputation and his discoveries.

So it is my belief that vulvar Lichen Sclerosis is a form of armoring due to a trauma or because the sufferer hates some aspect of his or her life, yet must continue in it because it is what is expected or required. *Ooh, you're thinking that the word "hate" is pretty harsh, right?* In my clinical experience most people (women in particular) are not comfortable using this word or owning the experience of it. So the body expresses it for us!

Let me acknowledge right now that I know that LS is not limited to women, but because I am a woman and because I've only encountered it clinically in women, from here on out, I am going to write as if you the reader, are a woman. My apologies to any male readers, and please know I appreciate you and mean no offence. Gentlemen, if you're reading this book for yourself, you'll still find lots of information to help you live happily ever after "*down under*" and if you're reading in order to educate yourself so that you can be a more compassionate and supportive partner, I take my hat off to you and say: Welcome & bravo!!

Now… isn't it terribly interesting where LS occurs most of the time? Yes, Lichen Sclerosis can occur on other parts of the body, but it rarely does. It mostly occurs in our nether regions… the parts we keep hidden and hardly even want to acknowledge that we have! In other words, there's likely some sort of sexual shame that goes along with this condition.

A year or so ago I came across Naomi Wolf's book titled: *Vagina* (2012, HarperCollins). (As a side note I recommend that anyone who has a vagina or anyone who has contact with a vagina should definitely read this book!) Ms. Wolf explains the newest science about the vagina but perhaps more importantly, she explores the cultural history of the vagina and the cultural inheritance that goes with having one. For example did you know that there is one word that is considered *"probably the most offensive and censored swear-word in the English language"; "the greatest slur"; "the most horrible word that someone can think of"; "the worst possible thing you can call anyone"; the word widely considered to be the most derogatory, the most violent, the most abusive".*

In case you are new to the planet… it's a 4 letter word that starts with "C" and rhymes with "hunt". And because I know so many women who are highly offended by this word, to honor them I'm not going to put it in print. But do you get it? Ladies, we all have one of these *"worst possible thing you can call anyone",* and just because you never use the word does not mean that you didn't inherit a belief system that compels you to act in a certain way so that you can avoid being labeled such a thing.

It's worth thinking about. Because if we don't consider how some of these cultural norms have affected and influenced us, we are limiting potential healing and our ability to move forward as a culture first, and as women second.

Understand that Ms. Wolfe uses the term *vagina*, not just in speaking of the opening to the womb (the "introitus" as the medical system calls it) but to describe any part of and the whole area – "from labia to clitoris to introitus to mouth of cervix." And I am doing the same, because LS can affect any of those external parts, and even the anus as we learned above. So ladies, I encourage you to think of the entire area as your vagina… the greater vaginal area or GVA (in geographical terms)!

Okay admittedly the "C" word is one of the less pleasant things that you'll read about in *Vagina* but trust me, it's an important read. For example you will learn about your "Incredible pelvic nerve", and how much of a woman's consciousness is tied to her vagina. That's right! Women think with their vaginas! There's even a pulsation that comes from this area, and if you focus on it, it will change depending on the situation you're in, and can even guide your decision making.

One of the crucial things you'll learn from reading *Vagina,* is that: *"Women are designed to receive pleasure, and experience triggers to orgasm, from* **skillful caressing and rhythmic pressure of all kinds over many, many parts of their bodies.** *The pornographic model of intercourse-even our culture's conventional model of intercourse, which is quick, goal-oriented, linear, and focused on stimulation of perhaps one or two areas of a woman's body - is just not going to do it for many women, or at least not in a very profound way, because it involves such a superficial part of the potential of women's neurological sexual response systems."*

Notice the part that I've bolded and underlined. When was the last time your lover involved any parts of your body other than your breasts and your vagina in your love making sessions? And who knew that they are supposed to? There really hasn't been an instruction book on this stuff! At least not one that's easily accessible to the average North American. But Naomi gives a beautiful guide in chapter 14 and in my opinion, it would be okay for a busy partner, to jump ahead and start with this chapter!

But for female LS sufferers, do read the entire book so that you can begin to piece the mystery together as to why you've developed such a debilitating and frustrating pathology in what should be your *sacred vagina.*

Notice what it feels like to think of that part of your body as sacred. Does it wake up a dormant part of you and make you feel strong and powerful? Or do you feel sad because you know that you have never been able to relate to that part of you that is sacred and powerful, and sexual?

It turns out that making love should begin 24 hours before penetration ever takes place. It involves looks, non-sexual touch, hugs (that position her nose near the armpit so that she can tune into her partner's pheromones) and affirmative, and loving talk that makes her feel confident about her attractiveness to her partner. All of this "foreplay" prepares the woman for the act of loving by calming her autonomic nervous system (ANS).

This is huge! How many of us have sex just to get it out of the way, or to get our partner to stop bugging us? What about make-up sex? Or even just sex to have a quick release so that we can get to sleep? This doesn't make us bad people, or our partners' bad lovers, but it is not serving us in a deeply spiritual, healing way. And it is likely involved in the LS pathology. So do yourselves a favor and read (at the very least) chapter 14 (of *Vagina*) so that you and your beautiful vagina get the message that you are a goddess and you deserve all of the pleasure that your vagina and your pelvic nerve were designed to provide you. When you choose to have sex, make it the kind that gives to you rather than takes from you, so that your vagina doesn't have to express the anger or sadness; shame or rage that comes from a sexual lifetime of (well) the North American model of modern sex.

And speaking of shame as related to sexuality, another highly provocative book to consider putting on your night stand is: *Sex At Dawn: The prehistoric origins of modern sexuality* by Cacilda Jetha' and Christopher Ryan (2010, Harper Collins). This book is really great for breaking thoughtful humans out of a certain "box" when it comes to thinking about sexuality. At the very least, it will force you to wonder where your particular "box" (read: beliefs about human sexuality) came from so that you can decide if they are true for you or not. Doesn't that sound healing!

In it you'll read about a traditional culture that was highly sexual in nature (sadly they've been gone for over 25 years now) where there was no un-planned pregnancy, ever! Imagine… these folks were extremely sexual and had no form of birth control, yet until a couple partnered off and had a ceremony, children were not conceived. Is it possible that unplanned pregnancies are the result of sexual shame? And if so, what other things might be the result of sexual shame?

You'll also discover that there are still Matriarchal cultures on this planet that consistently nurture confident, strong and sexually healthy individuals… something that seems to be a challenge in North America. It kind of makes sense when you consider that if no one knows who the biological father is of any of the children, the entire village takes responsibility for all children. Just imagine! You had a bad day at school but your mom is at work and can't listen and support you, so you head over to the next door neighbor's and they welcome you as their own and give you some hot chocolate and the compassion that you require in that moment. Heaven! (And no one is ever labeled "S-l-u-t" because there is no shame in owning and expressing sexuality in these cultures. Take a moment to imagine growing up without ever having known that word. What a different world for both males and females!)

Back to Wilhelm (Reich) again – in his book *The Murder of Christ*, we learn the true meaning of the story of Adam and Eve and more importantly, the meaning that our unconscious has run with and uses to create pathologies like Lichen Sclerosis. Do you remember the story? It doesn't matter if *you* do; your unconscious does! It's a story about being not only shamed, but damned and thrown out of paradise for your sexuality... all the worse if you're a woman because it was Eve who was seduced by the snake and then used her womanly ways to convince Adam to also taste the fruit from the (off limits) Tree of Knowledge. According to Reich the serpent was a symbol for LIFE and the "male phallus" (turned into a lowly reptile to be feared ever more, after its part in the downfall of man). The Tree of Knowledge was in the middle of the entire garden.

Let's think about that... in the middle of a garden (or life); in the centre of it all was one tree that God instructed Adam and Eve not to touch "lest ye die". If your body was a garden, what would be in the middle of it? And isn't it interesting that prior to partaking of the Tree of Knowledge, both sexes ran around naked. But magically they ate the fruit (don't you love the metaphors!), did not die but were suddenly stricken with shame and needed to cover their "private" parts. And then God punished them - BIG time!

Reich points out that to eat from the Tree of Knowledge is to know LIFE... and if you know life (or rather now you know how to make life) then you're

God-like, which seems to be what the bible is trying to prevent with shame and fear - Woman you had sex and as a consequence (for ever more) "In pain shall you bear children"!

Of course hormones eventually over-ride shame and fear (long enough for procreation to take place anyway), but the child born of a union riddled with fear of being damned out of paradise if caught, has some pretty big karmic baggage in him or her and will begat it and begat it and begat it.

And that's just your *unconscious* belief systems! What about the stuff that has happened to you in your life that you *are conscious* of and that likely contributed to belief systems that have helped to make you suffer in your genitals? Gadzooks it's staggering to think about.

But that's what this book is for… to make you think (because knowledge is power) and to offer you some simple tools (what to eat; what supplements to take; which Homeopathic remedies to help with symptoms) plus a pretty amazing tool (the Heilkunst system of medicine) that will tackle your past – ergo your false beliefs, so that **you CAN live happily ever after** "***down under***".

CHAPTER 2

Could your LS simply be a topical steroid addiction?

THIS IS AN important chapter and not a little provocative. And heck, maybe you won't need to read any further, after this one!

Think back. Have you EVER used a steroid medication for anything? I know I did. During my second pregnancy I developed a rash around my mouth (the typical place for "hormones" to show themselves on a woman's face) and when I complained to my obstetrician I scored a free sample of topical steroid cream. Then, after childbirth I was given a prescription steroid cream, to help my perineum heal. In fact, I stayed on that one off and on for years, as the area would get better and then a little worse after sexual contact. And I don't know why (maybe because my immune system was run down because of using a topical steroid for years and not knowing how to properly feed my body), but I eventually developed asthma and needed yet another steroid medication!!

But years later I learned that steroid use causes what is often diagnosed as eczema. And I am convinced that LS is an eczema-like condition.

Dr. Marvin J. Rapaport, M.D. has a wonderful video on youtube (https://www.youtube.com/watch?v=0JNVj6eAHDs&feature=youtu.be). In it he shares that he discovered Steroid Addiction (or "Red Skin Syndrome") years ago when he had a specialized practice dealing with the most difficult forms of eczema. Rapaport tells how other doctors would send him their most severe cases (of eczema) and after a battery of tests that all came back negative, it finally occurred to him that these people had used steroids for years and that the treatment was causing the eczema.

According to Dr. Rapaport the difference between a true eczema (which he says, usually runs its course by the age of 16!) is *burning*. Eczema itches like crazy but it does not burn. The burning sensation is caused from dilated blood vessels, which is what steroids do**. *Apparently steroid use anywhere on the body can cause these symptoms to show up anywhere on the body, even a place that you never put the steroids on!*** That means that if you had a little rash on your eyelid and used steroid cream on it for a few weeks, it could be enough exposure to cause Red Skin Syndrome (steroid addiction) somewhere else on your body. It travels 6 to twelve inches! And get this: the eyelids, armpits and groin suck the cream/ointment up faster than anywhere else, so the addiction or symptoms can happen pretty quickly in these areas. Did you catch that? The groin :O(

The cure for steroid addiction or Red Skin Syndrome is to stop the cortisone use. Period. Dr. Rapaport says that cutting back doesn't work because you'll eventually get another flare, which you'll also treat with cortisone and so on and so on. And sadly he says it can take a long time before the healing from the addiction is accomplished. In his practice they employ the use of powerful drugs to help people deal with the symptoms, as the addiction is dealt with (anti-itch meds, anti-inflammatories, and immune system suppressants) but he also recommends simple interventions like cool bathing, support from a friend or therapist and a wonderful and natural cream called Egyptian Magic that can keep the area moist while it heals.

But Homeopathy has a trick up its sleeve that MD's aren't aware of! Classical Homeopathy cures disease using the Law of Similars… *Like cures like (more on this in chapter 4)*. So your Heilkunst physician will treat for the disease state that's been caused by the use of the steroid with a Homeopathic dose (which is highly diluted) of cortisone applied in the appropriate potency(ies). At the same time Homeopathy offers other remedies to give relief of the symptoms. (For a list of possible remedies for symptom control refer to chapter 4 – *"Potions".*)

What was I thinking? Even if you have a steroid addiction that has given you a Lichen Sclerosis pathology, you do need to read on so that you don't suffer needlessly through the withdrawal!

CHAPTER 3

Blah, blah, blah just tell me how I can get some (right now) relief already!

ALRIGHT LET'S GET down to it! You want some relief, and this chapter is designed to help with exactly that. One caveat however: If you've skipped ahead to this chapter (and who can blame you, if you're in the midst of an acute, itch session that has you gnawing on the dog's rawhide bones!) please promise yourself (and myself) that you'll go back and read the rest of the book. There is a difference between relief and cure. And this book is designed to get you as close to cure as possible. (Is cure possible, you're wondering?) Well, in my practice I have seen it go away. The medical system says that it is not curable, so we won't call it a cure but relief, and even sending it away… those are the goals of this book. So read the whole thing.

As you've probably noticed by now, I love to give my readers a thorough understanding of everything mentioned in this book, and this chapter is no exception. But because I know some of you may really need relief, RIGHT now, I have put the recommendations at the beginning of each section in a larger font and in bold. That way you can skip the education until after the itch has settled down and you're better able to concentrate.

Basic Relief 101…

1. **Step away from the latte! And make today the last day that you eat (or drink) any kind of dairy.** Even organic and/or raw dairy will activate your immune system and can cause skin inflammation

because it has hormones in it that Mother Nature put there to make a little calf become a big cow really quickly. (Bonus: If you suffer from acne or rosacea this could solve that problem too!) You may notice improvement in L.S. symptoms in 2 to 3 days.

2. **Head to your local health food store and pick up a high quality Omega 3 fish oil supplement as well as an Evening Primrose one.** Each should be around 1000 mg's and commit to taking 2 of each daily, beginning today. You could feel significant relief in 3 days!

3. **Stop eating foods that cause inflammation, such as sugar, grains and alcoholic beverages.** Yes there is life (and a great one!) without regular consumption of these things, especially when you're free from LS symptoms. Changing your lifestyle this way, will make your whole body healthy, not just your genitals… and your waistline will thank you too!

4. **Consider if you could have a sensitivity or allergy to latex** and stop using it. This means condoms and diaphragms could be contributing to your condition, as could anything that you wear that has elastic in it. Stop the latex forms of birth control and consider going "commando" as often as possible to see if this changes your LS picture. (Of course you'll want to find another form of birth control… consider a google search of *Lady Comp* which is a little computer that has the same accuracy rate as the birth control pill! And in the meantime latex-free condoms are available.)

5. **Do a Tapping session (Emotional Freedom Technique) on the itching.** EFT is an amazing tool that you can use to feel a lot better! Head to the bonus section at the end of this book for a tapping script that can make you feel better right now.

Okay onto the lotions, potions and lasers (oh my!)…

Go to your MD and get a prescription for some topical cortisone cream or ointment (Please read chapter 2: *Could your LS Simply Be A Topical Steroid Addiction* as you weigh the pros and cons of this choice.)

And while you're waiting for the appointment go to a drugstore that carries the Bioderma line and buy some of their: **Sensibio Tolerance Plus. *With this stuff, you may be able to avoid the cortisone cream alto-gether!! (For more information on Bioderma's Sensibio Tolerance Plus, keep reading this chapter.)*

Okay but back to topical cortisone… many dermatologists prefer ointment for LS, so don't be surprised by this. Often the go-to choice for LS is Clobetasol.

I realize that some of you may be down-right shocked that I am recommending this. Before I address that however, I want to be clear that I am not talking to those of you who have been using topical cortisone treatment for your LS for weeks, months or even years already (these folks definitely need to read chapter 2, if they haven't already!). This recommendation is for the gal who is going crazy with the itch, and/or has the irritated, cracked, tight, burning and even oozing skin (because of scratching) that is making life unbearable.

What does topical cortisone cream do?
In a nutshell, it will stop the itching and help the skin to heal as long as you keep using it. But it does so at a price. You see your body is absolutely nothing short of miraculous. That's right! Even though you have a skin condition that's driving you bananas, your body is doing what it's supposed to… in fact that's why you have the symptoms. Here's how it works:

Your Life Force has identified some kind of problem; it may be purely physiological (but as a Heilkunst physician I can tell you honestly that there is no such thing as a purely physiological problem!) but more likely it is energetic in nature. For example let's say that you were not lucky enough to grow up in a highly functional family that spoke openly and honestly about sexuality and celebrated it. Nope, your family was pretty closed up (as many are) and ashamed of where babies actually come from. Your mother never really enjoyed sex and so she (unwittingly and largely unconsciously) passed on her beliefs around sexuality and the sexual act itself, to you. Then you had your first sexual experience. It was awkward, scary, exciting, painful, and (well) awkward! But low and behold, it even kind of re-enforced your beliefs about sex. Then you got into your first serious relationship. Turns out that guy had an anger management problem, and while the sex was furious and exciting at first (these guys think of sex as a hunting game... and you are the "prey") soon you were mostly only having sex after a huge fight.

Maybe you had a decent relationship along your journey, and things were nice but you guys just weren't meant to be, and then you met your husband. He's a great guy; the man of your dreams. The relationship is everything that you'd ever hoped for and the sex is great even, yet you developed this problem in your genitals.

First off, being in a great relationship can trigger healing. Why? Your body feels safe now, where it really wasn't in the right circumstances any time before.

And please understand what I am about to say: **You always get symptoms when you are healing.** That's really important to understand because it's very powerful. When you're in the midst of all-consuming itching, you're actually healing! That means you're not a victim!

For the body, this means that your immune system has mounted an attack. It has sent inflammatory chemicals to the skin around your vagina because it has sensed the "problem" and it is attempting to deal with it in the only way that it knows how. This is called "inflammation". Make no mistake, when your skin is red, hot, itchy, burning and cracked; peeling or flaking you've got an inflammation situation.

But our bodies have a natural anti-inflammatory on board. It's called cortisol. Natural cortisol is a hormone produced by your Adrenal glands and it controls inflammation. It is also part of the "fight or flight" response that your body activates when it perceives that you are in danger (or when your boss is yelling at you!). Cortisol (along with adrenaline) will cause symptoms like accelerated heart rate, sweating, anxiety and even weight gain around your abdomen (from too much exposure, over time).

Likely, *your* Adrenals have been a little over-worked (so many of us are trying to be Super-woman!) and your body is no longer able to produce enough cortisol to deal with the itch situation in your skin. Nope, your body is busy using the little bit of cortisol that it has left, to keep you alive.

Enter topical cortisone cream or ointment (steroids)! This synthetic version of cortisol (called cortisone) will do the same thing that your own cortisol does. But there is a down-side. Steroids over-stimulate your body, simply because we can't get the exact dosing down, the way your body brilliantly does. And so in time, the topical cortisone will actually cause your Adrenals to become more and more fatigued, meaning they will lose the ability to produce any cortisol.

And ladies cortisone cream or ointment is a steroid hormone. When you use it, your body responds by shutting down the production of its own hormone (in this case cortisol) because it recognizes that there's already some on board, so it feels it doesn't need to make more.

Additionally many LS sufferers have a Candida component to their pathology (see chapter 6). Candida is a fungus that we all have in our bodies but it needs to remain in balance or the symptoms are itching and irritation. Sound familiar? This fungus is put out of balance by a lifetime of too much sugar (in all of its forms... including grains) and genetically modified foods that are designed to destroy little critters in the environment (they destroy "good critters" inside of you and allow Candida to get out of control).

But Candida will also grow out of control because of certain medications – antibiotics, the birth control pill (FYI ALSO a synthetic steroid), and topical and inhaled steroids to name a few. So if using a steroid cream can cause Candida overgrowth then you can easily see another reason why this is neither a cure nor a long term solution to the LS situation.

This is where side-effects come into the picture. Side effects are simply the effects of a medication that you don't want or anticipate. So in the case of cortisone, we want the skin to stop itching and to heal. Unfortunately we can also get: itching and irritated skin from Candida overgrowth, burning skin, thinned skin, dependency (as the body produces less and less of its own cortisol), Tachyphylaxis (a diminishing response to the drug), changes to the menstrual cycle, thyroid dysfunction, fatigue, weight gain, thinning hair, etc.

Not a pretty picture! And one that I don't want you to develop, so please understand that the use of topical steroids is for desperate measures and that if you choose to go this route, then have all of the other suggestions in this chapter at the ready, so that once you've got this really nasty flare under control, you can employ other solutions to get you living happily ever after "*down under*".

Hot or Cold Pack (or Bathing)

I've known some women who sought relief from an acute attack of itching by putting a package of frozen peas on the area. **I do not recommend this and here's why:** As we've covered already, LS is inflammation. In simple terms this means that the cells in this area of your body are "on fire" and they are for a reason. Remember back in this chapter when I explained to you that symptoms are healing? Well as bad as inflammation is (and more and more research is showing that system-wide inflammation is responsible for many of our scariest diseases) it is a healing response.

So if you put out the fire (so to speak) with cold, you may find temporary relief but your body will respond by bringing it back, and it will likely be worse when it does. Not only that, it puts your body under further stress which can put you at risk for having your immune system go down and manifesting the latest "cold" or "flu" that you heard is going around. Believe me, it will take your body a ton of energy to recover from that cold pack (or cold bath), and then to re-inflame the area again. It's not worth it.

Now some of you may find that a warm or hot pack (or bath) really helps your LS symptoms, and that's great. This is the basic utilization of The Law of Similars! Your Homeopathic physician will be able to explain the Law of Similars further, but understand that when you apply heat to an inflamed area the body doesn't have to keep creating "fire", and so you can get some relief as it frees up some of its energy and calms down. It's worth trying, even if you haven't noticed that you are one of the gals who finds heat helpful. To review: **Heat is neat and cold is old!**

Consider a Red NaturaLaser

About a year ago one of my patients introduced me to Zero point energy products (zeropointglobal.com). She was doing very well in her Heilkunst healing journey but she had come upon these products and incorporated them into her healthy routine.

As I understand it, and as applies to the physical body, the Zero point is the perfect point that organ systems are at, when in a perfect state of health. I have simplified (or "Tammie-fied") that for my purposes so if you want more information on Zero Point energy, I encourage you to research it. It gets into quantum physics and such… fodder for another book – but not written by me!

The point is that these products are infused with frequencies that help to infuse our body's parts with the frequencies that they would be at, in a perfect state of health. That got my attention!

To be honest, while I only enjoyed playing with much of what I ordered from this company I did find an appreciable benefit from the Red NaturaLaser. Simply put, it works. I've used it on my face for break-outs, on tooth aches, on insect bites and even on the odd minor flare of LS. It gives instant relief to itching and burning. So in my book (oh look at that, this is my book!) it's worth putting in your LS tool kit!

Here's what I found on the website FYI…

"The Red Naturalaser Pointer has been energized and programmed with 60 essential Blueprint frequencies, primarily for the muscular system and skin. Our proprietary ZeroPoint technology delivers the protective field and balancing frequencies through one of the greatest carriers of frequency, light. In fact, light has been shown to be one of the most efficient conduits of energy ever harnessed. It's why fiber optic wire was chosen for the world's most critical communications platforms, sending pulses of information-laden light around the world in milliseconds."

One caveat here is that these products are sold by Multi-Level Marketing (MLM). For some (and you know who you are) that's an issue. Personally I've had my share of MLM experiences – some great and others not so great. But what's cool about MLM is that it gives people the opportunity to have a selling platform and to make some great money directly, by eliminating the costs of a "middle man". But (like any purchasing decision) you need to decide if this company resonates for you. Because I knew my patient well and was impressed with what she reported, I decided to go for it. I'm happy to report, that I am completely satisfied with my purchasing experience. (If you decide to purchase the Red NaturaLaser please note: I will not sell Zero Point products and do not benefit from mentioning them here.)

Salves, Creams & Potions

Maybe you've already considered this, but one day it finally hit me: I have super-sensitive, dry skin. I need 3 layers of goop on my face just to feel comfortable, so why don't I give my greater vaginal area the same consideration? I started making a morning and evening routine of putting salves, creams, etc. on my GVA. Some of them work really well, and sometimes I have to switch it up… just like on my face when the weather changes. See which ones work for you!

(Here's something that I learned the hard way - when you use most of the topically applied products listed in this chapter it will leave residue on your underwear! So you'll want to purchase underwear for daily use with your go-to happy ever after "down under" products, and extra undies for when you have your period, otherwise the adhesive on your 100% organic feminine hygiene products won't stick!)

Sensibio Tolerance Plus from Bioderma:

This is my most recent discovery and possibly my favorite. In fact, it's so great, that I've put it at the beginning of this chapter too! I found it at Shoppers Drug Mart here in Canada. I love this product because it seems to penetrate the skin and put moisture exactly where it is needed. My skin gets really uncomfortable, and has a tendency not to allow things in, but this goes in and makes my skin comfortable! Plus it is *designed for Intolerant or Allergic skin*. Here's what the website has to say:

"Reduces the hyperexcitability of the skin's nerve fibres and regulates the biological mechanisms responsible for the intolerance. The feelings of tightness and discomfort are soothed. The skin regains its original comfort."

I have checked the ingredients in this product and I feel that they are safe. Though they are not 100% natural or organic, the effect is amazing. And I am an extremely sensitive red-head remember. If I don't get an adverse reaction of any kind, the product is probably safe for most folks. That said, the next product has a similar effect and is extremely "clean".

Regenerating Day Cream by Dr. Hauschka:

Here's what the website has to say about Hauschka products...

"Both Dr. Hauschka Skin Care preparations and Decorative cosmetics are formulated with essences from medicinal plants grown biodynamically, organically, or responsibly harvested in the wild, using only the finest plant oils and natural essential oils

and are free from preservatives, artificial colors and synthetic chemical fragrances. By understanding the remarkable similarities between plants and the skin, special ingredients are selected to support particular skin functions, bringing balance by working in harmony with skin's natural rhythms. Since 1967, WALA Heilmittel, the manufacturer of Dr. Hauschka Skin Care, has produced pure, therapeutic and luxurious skin care. Biodynamically grown plants carry more vitality than plants grown by other methods. The gardens at WALA have been biodynamic for more than 40 years."

There's no doubt about it, the healthier the products you put on your skin are, the healthier you and your skin will be! Dr. H's Regenerating Day Cream also seems to penetrate the skin and bring moisture but it has a lot of botanicals, and us sensitive types can react to nearly anything at any time. I do love this product but some days, it just doesn't seem to provide the same level of comfort as the Sensibio Tolerance Plus does. And it comes with a hefty price tag. I get it! It's an amazing product, it's super-clean (and healthy for you and your world) and this "Regenerating" line of Hauschka products takes a year to make!! By the way, you should be using as many "clean" products on your body as humanly possible because what you put *on* your body, is going *into* your body. This particular company is one that I've been switching to month by month. So for those of you who can afford it, find a retailer in your area and try this "Regenerating" Dr. Hauschka product. Oh the price? I think I paid around $109 Canadian for the 40ml tube (don't tell my hubby!). But the Dr. Haushka brand has many products that are much more affordable so don't get turned off by the price of one cream.

Egyptian Magic: (check egyptianmagic.com for a retailer near you)
I learned about this product from Dr. Rapaport (chapter 2) and it is lovely. The consistency is similar to a barrier cream but it has wonderful ingredients that help to sooth, heal and protect the skin.

Ingredients: Olive oil, Beeswax, Honey, Bee pollen, Royal Jelly, and Propolis extract.

Clearly if you are allergic to bee stings or anything to do with bees, you'll need to avoid this product. But it's very interesting from a Homeopathic perspective (spoiler alert!!) because Apis Mellifica is a prime remedy for painful, itchy, red, inflamed skin (which I'll get more into in chapter 4) and it's made from the venom of a honey bee. So it's cool that this product helps on the outside, while a highly diluted dose of bee venom, will help heal the condition at the source.

The Dream Team: These 3 products were my "go-to" to keep my skin healthy and happy on a daily basis, especially as I was recovering from my topical cortisone use.

The first product in the team is: **Mint Matrix Oil Vera cream** from Zero Point Global. To really understand this product please reference what I've written earlier in this chapter about the Red NaturaLaser. But in addition to having the frequencies in it, this cream contains Aloe vera, Jojoba oil, Peppermint oil, Spearmint oil, Argan oil and Safflower Dulse. It is completely organic and is advertised to restore cellular balance from the inside out. Please note, that it is extremely minty. While the literature from the company says that it is safe to use on any orifice, if you've got a big LS flare that is raw and oozing, likely all that mint will really hurt at first. So go slow! But I found that adding just 1 drop to the other 2 products in the dream team was always the perfect amount.

Next on this list: **Nature's Essential Garden (Organic Multi-purpose) Jelly** (available at most health food stores) Yes, a safe and natural alternative to petroleum jelly! What's the problem with petroleum jelly? Well the first word in the name for starters. I like to avoid things that come from the petro-chemical industry as much as possible for health reasons and for environmental, as well as economic implications (why support Big Oil for anything other than what I absolutely have to?). But also because petroleum can contain breast-cancer-linked polycyclic aromatic hydrocarbons. In simple English that means it may contain an ingredient known to cause breast cancer.

Ingredients: Ricinus communis seed oil (Castor oil), Beeswax, Copernica's certifera (waxy substance from palm trees), Cocos nufifera (Coconut) oil and Tocopherol (vitamin E)

Another plus to this product (versus petroleum jelly) is that this jelly will help to get rid of fungus, as coconut is a natural anti-fungal. Petroleum jelly is an excellent barrier but it can create a wonderful breeding ground for fungus to thrive. Remember that Candida (fungus) is often one of the compounding issues that contribute to the LS suffering.

The final product in the team: **Kink-Ease MSM Salve** (www. stagesoflife.com). I learned about this product from reading Suzy Cohen's wonderful book: *Eczema, Itchin' For A Cure (www.suzycohen.com).*

Pharmacist Suzy Cohen, had a friend who suffered horribly from eczema and so she decided to write a book to help. What a great friend! Needless to say I highly recommend this read.

Suzy writes that some people are deficient in sulphur and that is why they get the symptoms of eczema. The symptoms she described sounded an awful lot like my symptoms so I decided to consider my LS eczema-like, and try some of her suggestions. To my great surprise this product often acts just like cortisone cream, in that it will stop itching and burning immediately! This may or may not be the case for you but it is certainly worth trying. There are a lot of ingredients, and I'm betting not all of them are "clean" but this is (according to Suzy) THE one MSM cream on the market that actually has enough sulphur in it to benefit eczema sufferers. (And on that note, MSM can be very helpful for sore, achy joints and muscles so feel free to rub it in any of those areas too.) *More about the use of crude sulphur later.

To use the Dream Team: Put a good amount of Jelly in the palm of your hand (about the size of a quarter); add (only) 1 drop of Mint Matrix Oil Vera cream; add a small squeeze of Kink-Ease MSM Salve; mix all three into a nice paste; apply to entire greater vaginal area.

Aloe Vera Gel: You'll find this extremely soothing, and fresh gel can really help with healing the area. Buy a plant and use the gel out of the leaves to get the full benefit (store bought is NOT the same). For a bad flare you can open a large leaf up and place it in your underwear like a sanitary pad.

*It is a good idea to keep the area clean. Many books and dermatologists suggest avoiding soap or using something like Dove. But Dove is full of chemicals that can irritate delicate tissue, no matter what the advertising says. A better bet is something from your health food store. Don't get anything fancy. Just find a soap that has pure, clean ingredients and that is formulated for eczema and/or very dry/sensitive skin. Watch out for ingredients like cotton seed oil. If it isn't certified organic it'll be loaded with pesticides and/or genetically modified for them, meaning it can be irritating or down-right harmful to not only your GVA but your whole body.

It is also recommended to avoid using a wash cloth or towel with LS. I think this is because the urge to scratch will be so intense. But in my experience, if your skin is doing well, gently using a washcloth daily, can help to remove dry, dead skin and will make it easier for the ingredients in the salves, creams or lotions to penetrate the epidermis and help several layers down. A towel is okay too, as long as you just gently blot. Suzy Cohen also tells us that **you should never apply anything to dry skin**… so leaving your greater vaginal area a bit damp, and then applying your moisturizer of choice, will make it easier to apply, as well as much more beneficial.

****Worth Mentioning…**

So, kind of like me and my story - where it took years and a major spiritually transformative experience for my LS to get better, I have one hold-out patient like that. Though the latest remedy (Platinum) is proving very promising indeed! However she has been savvy in her attempts to help herself, and recently started using **Lisepten Salve**, **Lisepten oil** and **Lisepten Tea**. She has kindly shared the link in case you want to try them too. Happily she has found great relief (at last!) from her itching and she credits these products. And with natural herbal ingredients like Comfrey, Calendula, Red clover, etc. it gets my seal of approval. Here's what the website says about the Lisepten oil:

"Herbs We Use & Why:

- *Comfrey: Heals skin tissues*
- *Calendula: Wound healer, anti-inflammatory, anti-fungal, antibacterial, antiseptic*
- *Red Clover: Anti-inflammatory, wound healer*
- *Lavender: Wound healer*
- *Plantain: Helps reduce itching, skin healer*
- *Chickweed: Helps reduce itching*
- *Witch Hazel: Antiseptic, astringent*

We add the herbs to almond, apricot, and sesame oils. The herbs steep in the oils, absorbing the healing benefits of the herbs. We then add 100% pure lavender essential oil which acts as a natural preservative as well as a natural wound healer. We also have a jojoba based salve which replaces the oils above with jojoba and sesame oils. This version is great for those with nut oil sensitivity. Refer to the related products section."

The Lisepten tea is facilitating healing of the gastro intestinal tract (from inflammation) so this combination is a good "inside-out" approach. Here's the link: www.cloverleaffarmherbsandgifts.com

One bit of caution is that we need to respect herbs as the medicines that they are. Yes, they are part of nature's pharmacy and much gentler than chemical drugs. But they often don't heal the underlying reason for a condition (similar to drugs), and over time you can also develop side effects from herbs just like you can from chemical medications. Additionally they can eventually stop having the same effect. So do your due diligence and keep working with the other suggestions in this book so that you can get as far on your LS healing journey as is possible for you!

**Don't waste your money…

There have been a few things that I've tried that didn't give any appreciable relief. I see myself as the "Canary in the coal mine", meaning that if it works for me and my red-headed sensitivities (while causing no harm), it will probably work for lots of folks. Ergo, if it doesn't work for me…?

1. Emu oil – if you google Lichen Sclerosis there will be lots of stuff that pops up about how people were miraculously healed from using Emu oil… specifically a brand that begins with a certain color. Don't be fooled, there is only one color of Emu oil, that color is just the brand name for that particular company! While Emu oil can be really great for the skin, (you can do your own research if you're interested) in my experience it doesn't penetrate the epidermis enough or really moisturize and facilitate comfort and healing below the surface, to bring any real relief for LS.

2. Alternative to cortisone creams (found in health food stores) – these are exactly what they sound like and for some people with mild skin problems, they may bring some temporary relief but I think that the list of herbal ingredients is a potential irritant to already super-irritated LS skin. In my experience they did not help at all, and exacerbated burning and suffering.

C H A P T E R   4

"Potions" (otherwise known as Homeopathic medicines)

Introduction to Homeopathy & Heilkunst

YOU'VE PROBABLY HEARD of Homeopathy before, but I'm guessing that until you picked up this book, you'd never heard of Heilkunst (H-EYE-L-Koonst). Well, *"Heilkunst is the original system of medicine that Samuel Hahnemann outlined in his Organon of the Medical Art (originally titled Organon der Heilkunst) which was a call for medical reform back in the 1700's! Samuel Hahnemann (1755 – 1843) is the "Father of Homeopathy" and the man whose genius brought us a system of medicine that actually cures disease, yet does no harm to the physical body."* (Taken from an article I wrote in the Mosaic Mind Body & Spirit Magazine in Autumn of 2009)

Heilkunst is THE system of medicine in its entirety and Homeopathy is a large part of it. *Homeo* means "same" and *Pathy* means "suffering". So this fancy word basically means this: If you want to give yourself a runny nose and eyes, then go cut up an onion. But if you already have these symptoms (because you have a cold or allergies), a Homeopathic dose of onion (a highly diluted dose) will stop them. And when I say highly diluted dose, I mean it! To make Homeopathic onion (Allium Cepa) a bit of onion juice would be put into about 9 drops of water and left to sit. Then one drop of that mixture would be added to 99 drops of water and alcohol and then shaken 100 times. This is a 1. To make a 2, you'd take a drop of the 1 and add it to 99 drops of water and alcohol, and shake 100 times. To make a 3, you'd take a drop from the 2 and so on, and so on. Now, when you get to a 12, if you were to take it to a lab for analysis (unless it's one of those super-crazy-sub-particle labs) they wouldn't be able to identify the original substance – the onion. Meaning that after 12, the dilution is so high that it is considered to be purely "energy" medicine. Essentially this means that Homeopathic medicines exert their action on the animating force (energy) in you that *gives* your physical body life, but not directly *on* your physical body. Many remedies that I prescribe on a daily basis are a 30c dose or a 200c dose so they've been diluted just as I've described, 30 times or 200 times. Isn't that amazing?! So now you see why this system of medicine can't harm you.

Ooh, I can hear your intellect firing up … That's ridiculous! There's nothing there! This girl is nuts! How can "nothing" do anything?!

But consider that Homeopathy was THE leading system of medicine worldwide until the birth of the American Medical Association. In 1855 the AMA added a rule to its code of ethics – called the "consultation" clause – that disallowed consultations with Homeopathic doctors and severely prosecuted any physicians who violated it. One poor fellow was really in a pickle, finding himself married to one! (Yep, he got kicked out of the AMA.) You can actually find the minutes of the meetings on-line! Here's one: *"We must admit that we never fought the homeopath on matters of principles, we fought him because he came into the community and got the business."* (*The Homeopathic Revolution* by Dana Ullman, MPH North Atlantic Books)

The rest of that sad story is that the AMA was largely created and funded by the Industrial Revolution. And part of that revolution was to make drugs on an assembly line, using bi-products of the petro-chemical industry. Energy medicine (by contrast) was/is made out of natural substances (like onions!) that can't be patented. No patent = no Big bucks!

By the way J.D. Rockefeller - one of the fathers of the Industrial Revolution and the richest man of his time - lived to the ripe old age of ninety-seven and was known to have his personal Homeopathic physician by his side, in all of his travels.

Leaving North America for the moment, and heading to the UK we find that the British Royal Family has employed its own Homeopathic physician(s) dating all the way back to Queen Adelaide (1792-1849). And there's no arguing how long-lived those royal ladies are!

Now as to the Heilkunst system of medicine, here's more from my article …

"Every shock or trauma that you've experienced throughout your life has left what Heilkunstlers call a "negative impression" behind. I like to think of these as old logs. When you're young, healthy and full of life, it's not such a big deal to carry around a few (energetic) old logs. But as the years go by and the traumas continue, you have to carry around more and more – that's not so easy. Eventually carrying around all those logs, leads to chronic disease."

So… Heilkunst employs the use of Homeopathic medicines to remove the negative impression(s) left behind by a lifetime of shocks and traumas, while at the same time teaching its patients how to take care of themselves through dietary and lifestyle changes. No topic is off limits and yes, we even talk to you about sex and orgasms (or the lack thereof, as the case may be ☺) plus other ways that you may need to improve on taking care of yourself.

Clear like mud?! Let's put it into context with an example…

Gloria is a 42 year old woman who's suffered with Lichen Sclerosis for approximately 6 years. She believes it began after the sudden and shocking death of her husband from a car accident. However she isn't exactly sure on the timing because "life was a blur for over a year after that" and because she's had issues with yeast and bladder infections for as long as she can remember.

(As an aside, Gloria recalls being very ashamed of her "larger than life" breasts in middle school and she remembers being afraid to be alone with her stepfather, once she had developed. She hates being alone generally and is currently in an undesirable relationship to avoid loneliness.)

After her husband's death Gloria was treated with antidepressants and she used alcohol and cannabis to self-soothe. There was an unfortunate night where she took a few too many anti-depressants combined with alcohol, which landed her in the hospital and a rehab program. She insisted that it had been an accident and that she didn't try to commit suicide, but no one would listen to her. She felt extremely violated and angry.

And most recently, her doctor prescribed pain killers and anti-inflammatories because she's been having pain in her back since she was "rearended" six weeks ago. Since starting these medications she's noticed that she's having a lot of stomach problems; she's gained abdominal weight; she's tired all the time and her LS symptoms have gotten worse. Because she hasn't found any relief from her medical doctor, she thought she'd try something else.

Generally a Heilkunst physician will follow the "map" of shocks and traumas from most recent, all the way back to your birth! In Gloria's case we would start with her most recent event (the medications and the car accident) and work backwards. However the death of her husband was a big shock to her. Her constitution (a Homeopathic term that basically means the one remedy that seems to fit her most with regards to her personality, her mind, her body/symptoms and her spirit) was really shattered by being suddenly left alone by her mate and it seemed to trigger an ongoing "victimization" disease state, which is likely why she (accidentally) nearly killed herself and then was locked up against her will. We can even see this in the nature of her recent car accident and in her choice to stay in a bad relationship to avoid loneliness.

To re-cap: In the Heilkunst system of medicine Gloria would be advised on how to make appropriate changes to how she is caring for herself (less alcohol/cannabis; more water; foods that heal her body instead of inflaming it; consider the relationship; etc.) and she'd be given support remedies for the presenting symptoms (constitutional dropper, physical pain, LS symptoms, as well as sadness/loneliness that is still ongoing since husband's passing), all in addition to being treated with ascending potencies of the appropriately chosen Homeopathic remedies to clear the left over negative impression(s) from each of the traumas we've identified above.

Here's the list of traumas (going backwards) that will be treated over the next several months...

1. Pain/Inflammation meds (also support her Adrenals as they are clearly fatigued – likely why the LS is worse, and begin Candida measures)
2. Car accident + Victimization
3. Anger/Frustration/Victimization from being forced into rehab (consider if #4 should be treated at the same time as this one)
4. Anti-depressants plus the alcohol that she OD'd with
5. Get more information on the year that was a blur (perhaps treat for the depression and prescribed meds as well as alcohol and cannabis)
6. Shock of her husband's sudden death (include: shock, grief, victimization and balance her constitution here)

Note: Because the death of her husband has been a Never Been Well Since (NBWS) event, it may be necessary to treat it much sooner than it appears on this well organized piece of paper! It may even be the first thing to treat. A good Heilkunstler always follows where the life force of the patient takes him/her.

...Okay here's my list of "Potions"...

The following are a list of some of the Homeopathic remedies that may help your Lichen Sclerosis symptoms. (The list could be endless but these are the ones found to be most effective in my practice/experience.) For a Homeopathic remedy to have the greatest chance of helping you, try to match the whole description to your personality, quirks and all symptoms, not just the Lichen Sclerosis skin symptoms.

**Please note that I STRONGLY advise you to consult with a qualified Homeopathic practitioner or (better yet!) a Heilkunst physician (heilkunstinternational.com). Yes, lots of health food stores do carry Homeopathic medicines but many people who've attempted to treat themselves are now the ones who say that Homeopathy doesn't work. You really do need to know what you're doing because the wrong remedy won't work, but that doesn't mean that the entire system is quackery. (Also keeping in mind what you've just learned about Heilkunst, these remedies will help with symptoms, but you'll still want to address the underlying reason for them in order to get a true healing or "Heiling"!)

Your Homeopathic physician will know exactly what potency to use, but generally a 30c (taken 3 times daily) is a good starting point. Keep in mind however, that the longer you've suffered with your symptoms and the more severe they are, the higher you may need to go. Potencies above a 200c are usually not available at health food stores.

Alumina: This remedy is made from Aluminum, which among other things is toxic to your nervous system. Consequently folks who may be helped by it can have mental dullness; an inability to hurry; difficulty in answering questions and they feel like they'll never get better.

Skin symptoms are dry (in fact all membranes are quite dry so there can be severe constipation) and generally worse in the morning. The symptoms are aggravated by heat. The itching can be quite intense and usually there doesn't appear to be any reason for the itch (no eruptions), yet this patient will scratch even to the point of bleeding.

Anacardium: People who need this remedy often feel like there's an angel on one shoulder and a devil on the other! And they don't know which way to behave, which is making them depressed and even considering suicide. Additionally these folks suffer from low self-confidence but they can also be hard and mean… or extremely angelic. All symptoms feel better after eating and there can be the sensation of a plug stuck in a spot of the body (like joints or stomach) and/or a sensation of a band around a part of the body.

Skin symptoms may include eczema and because this remedy is made from Poison Oak, it is helpful for tremendous itching that may be relieved by scalding water.

Arsenicum Album: People who may be helped by Arsenicum are generally fastidious, anxious, restless, thirsty for small sips, chilly and aggravated by cold. But their symptoms are generally better from heat. For these folks, there is a lot of burning sensation and the symptoms are often more on the right hand side of the body.

Skin symptoms are dry with intense burning and itching (yet feel better from heat). There may be a diagnosis of psoriasis or eczema and there can be ulcerations of the skin or no eruption at all. The itching is intense and it is often made worse by scratching.

Apis Mellifica: Made from honey-bee venom - "busy as a bee" we say, so people who may be helped by Apis tend to be active and busy all the time, though they are not thirsty. They also tend to get irritable, especially when challenged (and maybe they are a wee bit controlling). These folks are generally aggravated by heat and at 3:00 in the afternoon.

Skin symptoms include swelling, redness, heat and burning pains. Apis patients will be helped by cold applications and aggravated by warm/hot ones. They may have a diagnosis of eczema or hives which is quite swollen and feels better from a cold compress or soak.

Belladonna: This is one for the savvy homeopath to consider for LS symptom relief, especially if you think about some of the deeper reasons for the condition, as discussed at the beginning of this book (like rage or deep fear). Guiding symptoms for Belladonna's use are: Intensity, heat (so much so that you might feel it in your hand for a few seconds, after it's touched the affected area), scarlet redness, and cuts in the skin as though a little knife had been taken to it. Additionally the skin will be inflamed and can look pretty scary, almost like it's becoming gangrenous and (of course) there can be itching, swelling, burning, dryness and eruptions. Also, in my personal experience, this is THE remedy to consider when the itching is consuming all of your thoughts and making you crazy… or if scratching to the point of pain is morbidly pleasurable.

Calcarea Carbonica: If you're someone who's worked hard for way too long, has a strong sense of duty and responsibility, and is nearly so burnt out that you may have to take a leave, then this remedy might help your LS symptoms. Additionally, people who need Calc-carb can have a difficult time self-motivating and can be "fleshy" and "soft"; preferring a bowl of mashed potatoes or ice cream to chocolate. Calc-carb will help skin that's become "yeasty" (think about diaper rash), dry, cracked, itchy and red. And ladies if you've ever had a vaginal yeast infection or if you're prone to them, then think about Calc-c, as yeast (or Candida) may be part of your LS picture. (I'll get more into Candida soon!)

Calendula: A wonderful medicine which you can use in crude form topically, as well as in Homeopathic form to promote healing. (**Do make sure that any topical Calendula formulations are NOT mixed with alcohol, as this will dry and irritate your LS even more!) Think of this one if you've been scratching, because it will help it to heal so much faster than without. It also helps to control bleeding and sooth pain. Hmm, promotes faster healing, soothes pain and controls bleeding... sounds like the perfect remedy for the LS tool kit!

Candida: This is not typically a remedy found in a Homeopathic Materia Medica but it is readily found in Homeopathic Pharmacies and some health food stores. Using Candida in Homeopathic form is truly utilizing that amazing Law of Similars. So if someone is suffering from an imbalance of "Bad bugs" to "Good bugs," (Candida being a "Bad" bug) then a Homeopathic dose of Candida will help her body to get the Candida back in check.

Consider Homeopathic Candida if you suffer from the following: Vaginal yeast infections, rectal itching or urinary tract infections; athlete's foot or fungal infections of nails; skin problems like eczema, psoriasis, hives, etc.; digestive issues such as bloating, constipation or diarrhea; and chronic lethargy (to name a few). If these symptoms are part of your LS picture, then balancing Candida will be a big part of your relief. (Note, other measures will need to be undertaken and I'll cover those in chapter 6.)

Cantharis: This is often the first remedy that most Homeopaths think of for a urinary tract infection because it treats the intense burning pain associated with urination. It's also an excellent remedy (then) for relieving the pain of a severe burn and will help to facilitate healing of the wound. So you're probably getting an idea for why it can help the symptoms of LS.

This remedy is actually made from Spanish Fly – often mistaken for an aphrodisiac because the poison causes such intense burning and itching of the genitals that its victim looks crazed with passion! Perhaps that's enough said, but if your LS includes extreme burning and itching of the labia that's pleasurable to scratch yet brings no relief, *and* you find that you have "great anger and irritability" then Cantharis is a remedy for you to consider.

Causticum: This is a really important remedy for someone who seems to be suffering from "Sadness". But what sets this person apart from (say) a Natrum Muraticum type of sadness is that she has incredible sympathy for the suffering of others and gets really angry; even incensed over injustices toward herself or others (including animals). Her skin can be violently itchy, worse at night; tingling skin, swelling skin and ulcers that burn and have pus in them.

Cortisone: Here's another example of the Law of Similars. As discussed in chapter 2, many LS sufferers may actually have Red Skin Syndrome caused by past steroid use. So if you are suffering from a steroid-like disease, you need a steroid-like medicine to cure it.

Conversely I've found that a big part of Lichen Sclerosis is from Adrenal Fatigue. You see when your Adrenals are functioning optimally, they will supply your body with its own, wonderful anti-inflammatory (cortisol). And recall that LS is a condition of skin inflammation. So why isn't your body handling the problem with its own cortisol? Because chronic stress and other traumas have depleted the Adrenals so that they are more concerned with life support than skin conditions.

In the case of using a Homeopathic dose of cortisone to treat a steroid-like disease, the potency I find most effective to begin with is 30c. But for encouraging the body to balance its own cortisol I usually begin at a 7c dose, but often have to use a 5c in order to stimulate. You'll likely need your very own Homeopath in order to procure these potencies.

(FYI cortisone is the synthetic version of cortisol, which is what your body makes.)

Croton Tiglium: This remedy has an affinity for the skin *and* the intestines. For the skin, consider if you have small fluid-filled eruptions and if they are accompanied by "unendurable itching" particularly of the genitalia (and face). And if you do suffer from sudden, urgent diarrhea and loud rumbling and gurgling of your abdomen often, then these symptoms further indicate that this may be a remedy for you (probably with Candida).

Formica Rufa: Consider this remedy for intense itchiness that feels like there are ants running along your skin. Additionally your eruptions may resemble ant bites.

Graphites: This remedy is a wonder for when the skin has opened up, either from cracks or from scratching. Often there will be numerous sights of skin problems with cracks, but particularly where the skin meets the mucous membrane(s)… especially (but not limited to) if your problems are more on the left or began on the left. And here's an interesting guiding symptom: people needing this remedy can feel as if there are cobwebs on their face!

Histaminum: I've mentioned before that I believe LS is an eczema-like condition, and eczema can largely be triggered by foods that your body reacts to by producing Histamines as part of the inflammation. You've likely heard of antihistamines (and maybe even used them in a pinch!) like Benadryl? Well here is the Homeopathic alternative to those chemicals!! Again, utilizing the Law of Similars, when we give the body a highly diluted dose of what's causing the itching and swelling, it can stop it in its tracks.

Hura: This remedy is made from latex. So if you are sensitive to or allergic to latex, or if you think it may be irritating you then this remedy will help you heal from it.

Even if you don't have an actual physical problem with latex, consider Hura if you feel intensely hopeless and like you don't have a friend left in the world, in addition to your skin problems. *Hint, when this remedy is needed you might find yourself obsessively checking a mirror to see if you look alright or if any blemish has gotten worse.

Hypericum: This is a wonderful remedy for helping with pain, particularly if it is sharp and/or shooting pain and especially for parts that are rich in nerves like the tips of your fingers, your teeth and your genitals.

Kreosotum: This is probably THE remedy most utilized to deal with a vaginal yeast infection. While it does treat the itching that comes from a discharge, it may or may not help your LS symptoms if they are not currently related to a yeast infection. But if Candida *is* part of your LS picture or if you are currently suffering with an itchy discharge that may be putrid and causing sores and or swelling of your greater vaginal area, then Kreos can work miracles. It probably goes without saying, but the guiding emotional symptoms for Kreos are irritability and a fear or aversion to sex. (Nobody feels happy or sexy when she has a yeast infection!)

Lilium Tigrinum: This remedy is considered to be the "Most irritable of all remedies". So not only is the gal who needs Lil-tig super-rage-filled, but she can have a crazy or "wild" feeling in her head and she's always rushing. She may even find that she can get into a state where she's full of sexual excitement. And while she may or may not act on this, she also has a deeply moral/religious state to her and the see-saw between feeling extremely sexually excited and extremely moral is what makes her reach a frantic state. You can just imagine how "crazy-making" that would be, even to the point of feeling suicidal. Her skin can be: tingling, burning, itching and may even feel like insects are crawling on it (formication). Lil-tig folks may resort to self-torture for relief of the mental state (think: cutting).

Medorrhinum (Called Sycosis in Hahnemann's time): This remedy is often very important in treating LS because it can be part of the underlying reason for the disease. You see Medorrhinum (Med) is what Samuel Hahnemann (The Father of Homeopathy) considered a Chronic (long-lasting and difficult to eradicate) disease – termed "Miasm". During his time, he identified three such chronic Miasms and in my experience this one and Psorinum (coming up) are the two most well indicated for Lichen Sclerosis sufferers. What this means is that to give you the most successful treatment, likely you'll need one of these two remedies (or even both) along with some of the others on the list, to treat the symptoms of these two. Keep in mind that all beings suffer from Chronic Miasms and the various events we experience as shocks or traumas in our lives, will turn the symptoms of them on.

People who will likely benefit from adding Med somewhere in the treatment of LS may have a history of "extreme" behavior or emotions. For example they will have THE worst diet one day, and then become vegan the next. They may "need" alcohol or recreational drugs on a regular basis and these gals likely suffer from spring-time allergies. Her symptoms may have begun after a new sexual relationship started and she can have a history of herpes and/or genital warts. Inflammation of any kind is part of the Medorrhinum picture (so arthritis sufferers with LS should be considering Med).

Skin may be scaly and patchy, hardened; eczema; warts; warty growths (can be black in color) and worse on right; herpes, acne that is large, red and angry; yellowness of skin; intense and incessant itching often better at night; itching can be worst on back, vagina and labia and is made worse by thinking of it; vaginal discharge (if there is one) is usually green(ish), excessive, and can smell of fish.

Mezereum: A big remedy for skin problems. Consider it if you often feel anxiety in your stomach and if you tend to be chilly and aggravated by cold. And this is interesting… the person needing Mez can have an extremely sensitive scalp, even too sensitive to be touched, plus there may be a lot of skin problems on the scalp.

Skin problems usually begin with intensely burning/itching cysts which crust or thicken after scratching. The itching is made worse by heat and by being in a nice, snuggly bed but may be helped by an application of cold. Also consider for skin that cracks, especially if there is a geometric pattern to the cracking, or for when there is itching yet no appreciable eruptions.

Natrum Muraticum: In school we learned to think of the little donkey named "Eeyore" from the Winnie The Pooh stories, when we studied this Homeopathic disease. She tends to be overly serious and proper, perfectionistic, gloomy, averse to company, and very much affected by grief. If you think back and realize that your LS began after your lover left you (or even after a temporary break), this may well be a BIG part of healing for you. The skin symptoms for Nat-m folks are itching, prickling and stinging. There can be tiny eruptions over the entire body and generally eruptions are dry and can be cracked. The genitals can be itchy; there can be an aversion to sex and sex can be painful because of dryness of the vagina but she can also have a dry mouth and dry skin. Also think of Nat-m if you suffer from migraine headaches *and* LS, especially if the headaches are made worse by light, sun, reading, noise, and before or after your menstrual period.

Petroleum: Another BIG remedy for skin problems. (And especially think of this one if you work with tar or petroleum chemicals – Hairdressers, this means you!)

If you've got super-dry skin and it seems like there hasn't been a cream or lotion invented that will penetrate it, this is the remedy to consider! Skin can have deep cracks that may be bloody. Itching can be so severe that you scratch until your skin is raw, and that itching is often worse at night and worse from being snuggly warm in your bed. You may have been diagnosed with eczema, psoriasis or herpes and generally speaking your skin problems seem to be worse in the winter, better in the summer.

Phosphorus: This gal is the fun one who everyone wants to hang out with! She's exuberant, dramatic, effervescent and maybe a little gullible. She can also be quite sensitive to her world, especially to people's energies, odors and environmental toxins. She NEEDS some alone time to re-charge (but may be anxious from being alone for too long). Symptoms for this gal tend to be worse on the left side and skin is dry, possibly with a psoriasis or eczema diagnosis. Itchy skin is worse at night and worse from heat. Her symptoms may be better from rubbing the area and from eating or sleeping.

Platinum: If vaginal penetration has become challenging for you (because of muscular contractions not your skin symptoms) then consider this remedy. An interesting state of mind to watch for is the idea that you are somehow "above" everyone else. You might think you're more advanced spiritually or that you always take the moral high ground where others don't, or maybe you've (secretly!) always imagined you were somehow descended from a royal family. You're likely very passionate, and others may find you rude and self-absorbed (be honest with yourself; this is for you and no one else).

Your GVA will be extremely over sensitive and likely you feel a lot of heat and itchiness in the area. Even the slightest touch may make you sexually aroused; conversely an increased sex-drive or sexual excesses can also be a guiding symptom for Plat. Also if you have the sensation that a band is wrapped around any area of your body, this is a strong indication for Plat too.

Psorinum: Samuel Hahnemann called this "The Mother of Disease". It is the 2nd Chronic Miasm on our list, but only because I've listed them in Alphabetical order. Dr. H. taught that all disease originated from this one.

And for folks who suffer from skin issues, we kind of get a hint right in the name: Psorinum ...psori-asis. Coincidence? Nope.

When a gal is very pre-occupied with lack (of money) then likely this remedy is part of her solution. That "lack" can spill over into many aspects of life and will often manifest as not enough moisture, so the skin and mucous membranes are quite dry for her. She's often not warm enough either and may find that she must cover her head all year long. Psora can cause intense carb cravings too, and all symptoms are generally worse in autumn. She can get eruptions on her genitals and her skin itches horribly. The itching is worse at night and from being over-heated or being warm in her bed. Often she will scratch until she bleeds and she won't sleep from the itching. There may be a history of Scabies and it can be recurring. Virtually any skin condition can be in this Miasm... boils, warts, oily skin, acne, eczema and yes - psoriasis.

Pulsatilla: This remedy is known for its changeability. For example the gal needing Puls may find that she changes her mind a lot, that her menstrual cycle is never the same twice, and that her bowel habits change every day! She is also known to be quite sweet among her companions and when she is under the weather (physically or emotionally) she really needs company to feel better. She is warm yet not very thirsty and can suffer with a vaginal discharge that is thick like cream and can be irritating and burning particularly if it happens before, during or after her period.

Skin symptoms can be changeable too but if there's itching it'll generally be burning or prickling and it'll be worse in the evening, at night, and from the heat of bed. And Pulsatilla's itching gets worse the more that she scratches. Some ladies find that they get little black spots from scratching. If your doctor has said these are nothing to worry about then likely they are a tiny kind of varicose vein and this remedy may be the one to help if the other symptoms match for you.

Radium Bromatum: In case you happen to be someone who's had a lot of X-rays in your life, this is a prime remedy for you to consider. But

even if you haven't, you should still consider it. The person who needs it is generally warm-blooded and will be aggravated by the heat of her bed and by night in general. Problems can go right to left or left to right. Skin symptoms may be diagnosed as eczema, psoriasis or even ringworm. Eruptions are dry and burning and may be over the thighs and genitals; there can be persistent itching of external female genitalia.

Rhus Toxicodendron: I bet you can't guess what this remedy is made from? Of course you can't from the name – unless you speak Latin?! It's Poison Ivy! If you've never had it, read on. Actually read on even if you have…

Rhus-tox may help you if you're the type of person who is always cheerful and joking, but restless (restless especially in bed). However you may be irritable, impatient, hurried, and quite superstitious. And maybe you crave cold milk. This person is actually made worse from cold weather or cold bathing but feels better from warm weather and/or bathing. Symptoms are often left-sided, usually worse in the morning, on getting up and worse in the autumn. Consider this remedy if you have painful but especially stiff joints, in addition to your LS symptoms. (Or even if you're a tiny-bit "inflexible" in your thinking.) The skin symptoms are intensely itchy but better from scalding hot water. Skin conditions it can help include eczema, herpes, shingles, poison oak or poison ivy, hives or psoriasis. And if your skin has been problematic for a long time and has become thickened, this is a good one to consider.

Rhus Venenata: You can consider this remedy if you have the skin symptoms of Rhus-tox but none of the joint pain/stiffness, nor the craving for cold milk. Unlike Rhus-tox, this remedy has a lot of prominent cracking of the skin and terrific itching. Itching is worse in the evening, in a warm room and in bed. And after scratching and rubbing (which is irresistible!) the itching is intolerable. Especially consider this remedy if your LS is causing you anal symptoms such as intolerable itching and burning and/or neurologic pains there.

Sulphur: This is probably the first remedy that anyone who knows anything about Homeopathy, thinks of for a skin problem. And with good reason! Especially if Psorinum is part of your picture, then Sulphur could be a great one to help you too. Folks who may be helped by Sulphur can be full of energy and may have a bit of a reputation with their families for being messy and/or lazy. However Sulphur females tend to be quite business-minded or the one family member who is beautifully organizing and managing – well, everything! Loose stools can often be a guiding symptom for Sulphur, especially if it's first thing in the morning and sends you running from your bed to the bathroom. Sulph tends to be quite warm and can be aggravated by heat and she is quite bothered by odors… especially the body odor of others, but she loves her own :O)

Skin problems are usually moist and itch horribly. And the itching gets worse from heat, the warmth of bed, at night in general, from bathing (in fact if you're not too fond of bathing consider this remedy!) and from wool. Nearly any skin problem may be helped by Sulphur but especially ones with a terrible itch.

What about an actual crude dose of sulphur?

Sulphur is an essential nutrient – a mineral. It plays some important roles in maintaining the health of your body. In fact you may have heard of supplements like Chondroitin sulphate or Methylsulfonylmethane (MSM) for joint health. Even an Epsom salt bath is supplementing with sulphur! Sulphur is found in over 150 compounds in your body. Sulphur components are in nearly every type of body cell and in many of the foods we eat… meaning that it's vitally important.

Why am I telling you this? Because sulphur was part of my healing journey and it may be part of yours too. (Hint: if the Kink Ease MSM Salve helps your symptoms then definitely read on about taking crude sulphur!)

Once I learned Homeopathy, every time things became unbearable I'd repetorise my symptoms *again*. That means that I'd go through the process of figuring out which Homeopathic remedy would be the best one to help my symptoms. Sulphur was the one that always showed up as #1. But EVERY time I took it, I'd get worse… way worse…unbearably worse. As a homeopath I know that getting worse can be a good thing, but only if it's followed by getting better and it never was for me. (*Though I've used Homeopathic Sulphur many times in my practice for others, and it works beautifully!)

But at some point on this amazing healing/spiritual journey I made a discovery. One leg of the journey had taken me to the Hawaiian island known as The Big Island. And while I was there, my LS symptoms significantly improved… as I (somehow) knew they would. But a few months later, they began to come back. You can imagine how devastated I was. Why? What was I doing wrong? What changed?

The good news about desperate ruminations is that sometimes they actually bring clarity! I was racking my brain attempting to figure out what was different and why things were going backwards. Idyllic paradise? Check. Was I relaxed there? Check. Did I eat differently there? Not really. Did I take my supplements there? Yes, that hadn't changed. Was I in the sun more? As a fair-skinned red-head… No! I did drink more coffee there. Hmm.

The Big Island is known for its Kona coffee. Any coffee lovers out there probably know that it is fantastic coffee, because it grows on the slopes of Hualalai, an active volcano. (No, I'm not telling you to drink more coffee so keep reading!) I confess that I hadn't been too fascinated with the volcanoes while visiting the island but I now wondered if being in an environment with active volcanoes might be part of my LS puzzle.

Then it hit me – sulphur! (*Please note that I've made the distinction between Homeopathic Sulphur and the mineral sulphur with a capital S or a lower case s wherever possible.) I'd been in an environment with a lot more sulphur than anywhere else I'd ever been. Because of the active volcanos it was in the food, the air, the coffee! And elsewhere soil depletion is a very real problem, with sulphur being one of the depleted nutrients. So I began eating more sulphur-rich foods (like egg yolks, garlic, onions, Brussels sprouts, cabbage, broccoli, chicken, fish and yes, even coffee). I also took a supplement of MSM and/ or garlic. I'd alternate between the two. You can also absorb sulphur from Epsom salts baths and you may find it soothes a bad LS flare. In fact, later I discuss what the herbicide Glyphosate is doing inside your body and crude sulphur can be very helpful for helping to heal that problem too!

(**As a side note, dairy has sulphur in it too and I did increase my organic dairy consumption at that time. However, I've since confirmed that dairy added to my symptoms and is largely implicated in skin problems of all kinds. With the added sulphur my symptoms were about 85% improved but when I took out dairy a year later, it got me to 99.8%!)

But because I'm a Homeopath I also took a dose of Sulphur 6c. And it made me better, not worse! Why? Because a 6c is a dose that still has some actual sulphur in it. It's a dose that's designed to encourage your body to take in or create more sulphur whereas the 30c or 200c (or higher) doses of Sulphur I'd taken in the past, were to treat a Sulphur-like disease state. My body didn't like that! It wanted MORE sulphur, not less. That's what it had been trying to tell me with the symptoms and why the repertories always came up with Sulphur! I can't tell you how blessed I feel to have understood this, and how happy I am to share that with others who may benefit from my experience!! Keep it in mind and discuss it with your health care provider as you plan your own healing journey. (Or go to Kona and test for yourself!)

Thuja: If you feel that if people really knew you, they wouldn't like you, or if you identify with words like: brittle, breakable; fragile then Thuja may be for you. Also think of this remedy if you have had problems ever since a vaccination, or series of vaccinations. An interesting symptom of Thuja is that women can be extremely afraid of pregnancy but there can be a feeling that something is "alive" in the abdomen. And for fear of being hurt, they don't want to be touched. Additionally if you have a sweet smelling sweat, particularly in your genital area, then it is well indicated. The vagina will be super-sensitive too, making intercourse painful and the sensation afterwards is like being bruised. There may be a diagnosis of eczema or psoriasis so itching, cracking, burning, etc.

Urtica Urens: This remedy is often used to treat first and second degree burns so if your LS symptoms include burning, consider it. It is an excellent skin remedy especially for burns, hives and eczema and for itching or swelling of the genitalia. There's not a lot to go on for the state of mind of Urtica Urens but the books say: "Terribly giddy". (That said, the last time I had a sun burn I needed this remedy and I was actually pretty grumpy.)

> ****Note to practitioners:** As you continue through the Heilkunst journey with your LS patient, likely you'll need to treat the Miasms: Carcinosin and Syphilinum at some point, though they are not listed here as acute symptom help.

**Don't be afraid to combine remedies (but preferably with the help of a qualified practitioner!). Sometimes one remedy will nail all of your symptoms, but that is pretty rare. When I was in Kona (a place on The Big Island in Hawaii) the following combo came into my consciousness. It was just another step on my spiritual/healing journey but it was an important one, as it gave that much more relief to a situation that had debilitated me for years.

Tammie's Kona Combo: Cantharis, Phosphorus, Belladonna, Calendula, Alumina, Rhus Venenata

Let's look at the parts to this informed combination of Homeopathic medicines…

Cantharis – I suffered with a terrible burning pain, the area looked like it was perpetually burnt and was extremely sensitive to any touch/contact.

<u>Phosphorus</u> – When you begin working with a Homeopathic physician you'll learn about your constitution. Basically it is YOUR remedy that when taken, will strengthen your entire person (mind, body and spirit). This is my constitutional remedy.

<u>Belladonna</u> – My symptoms were extremely intense and sometimes all consuming. As I described at the very beginning of the book, I could suddenly become crazed and scratching was morbidly pleasurable. Plus the area always looked cut, red (a big key-note of Bell) and heat could be felt radiating externally from it, while I would feel the blood pulsating internally.

<u>Calendula</u> – This is such a comforting, healing remedy! It's like Chicken Soup for The Skin.

<u>Alumina</u> – As I've mentioned already, my GVA (and all of my skin) can be exceedingly dry and this is one of the key remedies for dryness of all membranes. But it also has itching of skin with no visible eruption and scratching to the point of bleeding. So it was a great choice for my particular symptoms.

<u>Rhus Venenata</u> – Both Rhus-tox and Rhus-ven fit my itching symptoms but this one also has cracks in the skin. So for that difference and because I didn't suffer with joint problems, Rhus-ven was the better choice for me.

So you see, my Lichen Sclerosis symptoms were not just one Homeopathic disease state, they were six! (And that's not including the Chronic Miasms under the symptoms.)

Trying only one remedy for a long-standing, intense problem with multiple symptoms can be another reason why some people have been falsely led to believe that Homeopathy doesn't work. But understand, this chapter is only about symptom control. It is important to follow all of the recommendations in the book to get as close to cure as you can get… meaning to fix the reason for the symptoms in the first place!

CHAPTER 5

Daily Housekeeping for living happily
ever after "down under"

WHAT I'M ABOUT to say may shock you, but stay with me... North Americans bathe too much! Yep, we do. And in addition to adding to the depletion of a natural resource (fresh water), we are depleting the natural (healthy) bacteria on our skin. The more you do that, the more unhealthy critters have a chance to grow and thrive on your skin. So consider taking a shower or bath only once or twice a week. And use "clean" products much like your great-grandparents would have used. We don't need to use chemicals and the idea that we should be "squeaky clean" was just an advertising campaign that we all bought into. (Consider companies like Annmarie Skin Care, Intelligent Nutrients, Mercola.com, Natural News, Morocco Method, Dr. Haushka and Eminence for "clean" hair and body personal care products.)

What I keep in my bathroom is a good, old fashioned basin (you find them in antique stores now). I fill it up with tepid water and I wash the parts of my body that can get a little stinky. (By the way squatting over the basin is great for your back, as well as helping to strengthen your pelvic floor muscles!).

Keeping the area clean: Here's a reminder from chapter 3 about washing your greater vaginal area...

"It is a good idea to keep the area clean. Many books and dermatologists suggest avoiding soap or using something like Dove. But Dove is full of chemicals that can irritate delicate tissue, no matter what the advertising says.

A better bet is something from your health food store. Don't get anything fancy. Just find a soap that has pure, clean ingredients and that is formulated for eczema and/or very dry/sensitive skin. Watch out for ingredients like cotton seed oil. If it isn't certified organic it'll be loaded with pesticides and/or genetically modified for them, meaning it can be irritating or down-right harmful to not only your GVA but your whole body."

And if you're having a bad flare, you'll want to do as little as possible to the area, but still feel clean. Coconut oil to the rescue!! You can use it to wash with (it won't lather and it won't completely rinse off) and just rinse with tepid, clean water. Or in a pinch you can take a handful of it, make sure it's emulsified and spread it over your entire GVA. Then use toilet tissue to gently wipe, as you would after going to the bathroom. This will moisturize and deodorize the area, plus coconut oil is anti-inflammatory, anti-fungal, and anti-bacterial, meaning that it'll soothe the area *and* keep you clean.

After cleansing moisturize the area (see chapter 3), but if you've "washed" with coconut oil you may not need any additional moisture. Pay attention so that you'll get to know your GVA's particular needs. By the way, feel free to use coconut oil as an intimate lubricant for sexual activity (though confirm its safety with the condoms you use) or if you're suffering from vaginal dryness.

And speaking of wiping after going to the bathroom, I'm sure your mother taught you to wipe from front to back but did she also teach you to use a pre-moistened "wipe" too? This has become fairly common place but I urge some caution here. First off, those wipes can be loaded with chemicals that simply aren't good for your GVA skin or for the rest of you. And please don't flush the wipes no matter if the package says that it is safe to do so or not! This is becoming a really big problem for many cities in North America. However, I am an advocate of thoroughly cleaning the "back of the bus" after a bowel movement but I recommend 100% organic, cotton rounds. Yep, the same things that you use to clean your eye makeup off! All you need to do is wet them (probably three), wring them out and then carefully use them to clean the area. (Then toss in a covered garbage.)

Admittedly rounds are a little less convenient than wipes but your health is worth the bother. You'll find that things are a lot more sanitary back there, and that if you do suffer from anal itching, this can significantly help that problem.

(Also from chapter 3…) "It is also recommended to avoid using a wash cloth or towel with LS. I think this is because the urge to scratch will be so intense. But in my experience, if your skin is doing well, gently using a washcloth daily, can help to remove dry, dead skin and will make it easier for the ingredients in the salves, creams or lotions to penetrate the epidermis and help several layers down. A towel is okay too, as long as you just gently blot. Suzy Cohen (*Eczema, Itchin' For A Cure, www.suzycohen.com*) also tells us that **you should never apply anything to dry skin**… so leaving your greater vaginal area a bit damp, and then applying your moisturizer of choice, will make it easier to apply, as well as much more beneficial."

Underwear: By now your doctor has likely told you to wear white, cotton undies only. And that's good advice, especially if you can find 100% organic ones. Cotton so that the area "breathes" (making it more difficult for organisms like yeast to get out of control) and white because many people will have a reaction to the chemicals used to turn your undies into all the colors of the rainbow.

I also like bamboo underwear and I especially like ones with a simple band around the legs. The less lace, frill and elastic, the more comfortable they will be. Save the sexy ones for a "special night" once your "*down under*" is nice and happy! (Except for thongs. They are a definite "Don't!" Sorry ladies, but thong underwear and a healthy GVA are natural enemies.)

Laundering your "delicates": For ladies suffering with any kind of "*down under*" issues my tried and true method for laundering your undies goes like this:

1. Have a lot (like 22 pairs) so that you can do one load of undies every few weeks.

2. Wash your undies in hot water.

3. Make sure that the soap you use is toxin and chemical free, and designed for super-sensitive skin, and use VERY little.

4. Do not use fabric softener, but you can use some vinegar if you like (it will soften the fibre in the fabric as well as kill fungus like yeast/ Candida).

5. Add a few drops of liquid Grapefruit Seed Extract to the detergent dispenser (also a great way to kill any extra "critters" you wouldn't want living in your undies like Candida).

6. Make sure all underwear is dried thoroughly and DO NOT USE DRYER SHEETS! Up until now, if you have been using dryer sheets you may want to invest in a new dryer and stop it. Seriously! Do you have any idea how many chemicals are in dryer sheets? Not only are they irritating to your sensitive skin but the emissions out into the environment are toxic. If you currently can't afford a new dryer, then stop using dryer sheets anyway, and at the least, hang your undies to dry from now on.

Toilet Paper: This may be something that hadn't occurred to you but it can be a big part of the LS picture. There are toilet papers available that are tested to be less allergenic than others. Of course this isn't a guarantee, but they are worth a try. And do be sure not to use any colored varieties, just like with your undies! (Cashmere was my "go-to" brand until I discovered Bamboo toilet paper (BTP)... see below.)

But I've recently discovered toilet paper that is made from Bamboo and I'm definitely a fan! My #1 reason is because there is no BPA in many of the Bamboo toilet papers. This is another nasty chemical and one that mimics the hormone estrogen. Because of modern industrialization most of us have way too much xenoestrogen (fake estrogen) already, so wherever you can avoid it, I recommend that you do. The other reason I love "BTP" is because it doesn't leave any of those tiny bits of toilet paper behind after wiping. Those little pieces (that no one seems to talk about!) can get stuck in/on super-dry, irritated skin, and they only make things worse. That problem is completely eliminated by the bamboo paper. And you can feel good using it because bamboo is completely environmentally friendly. Trees take 20 to 50 years to be mature enough to make paper products out of, but bamboo is usually ready in only 4 years. So really: Buy BTP and save a ton of trees :O) One caveat however, is that if your skin is really sore, and/or fissured, this may not be the time to use BTP as it isn't the softest toilet paper. One like Cashmere (the name says it all but no, it's not made of cashmere!) will be better for you until your skin is feeling better.

Okay so we've talked about intimate wipes, toilet paper and thongs - we might as well talk about poop…

Constipation could be adding to your Lichen Sclerosis suffering. How? Think about all that straining and rocking back and forth. That's putting a lot of physical wear and tear (literally) on your delicate tissue. So if constipation is an issue for you (stool is too large or just never gets completely pushed out), talk to your health care provider about becoming a *healthy* eliminator. Often the problem in women is a simple magnesium deficiency (not to mention fibre and water!) but your practitioner will help you to determine the best course of action for you. **Laxatives are okay for occasional use, but any more than that will cause a dependency and actually exacerbate the problem (yes, even herbal ones from your health food store).

Feminine Hygiene Products: Years ago there was an issue with women getting sick and even dying, from wearing tampons for too long. That's why the recommendations to change them more frequently came out. But the real problem was what the tampons were made out of. If you're putting synthetic fibres into your body or cotton that's been heavily sprayed during growing and then chemically bleached to be snow white in color (super-ironic for tampons and pads. I mean seriously, why not just dye them red?!), then you're exposing yourself to toxins via your vagina. And it will absorb them. Even if you're not using tampons, please, please, please make sure that your pads are made from reputable companies that use 100% organic cotton. It's healthier for you and for the environment and definitely gentler on your LS skin. You may even consider using washable pads, but if you have a heavy period, this will be a lot of extra work and you'll want to make sure you're careful about how you wash them in a non-toxic way.

Polyester, Pantyhose & Jeggings: In case you haven't already made the connection, many of your personal style choices could be exacerbating your LS condition. Anything that is tight and/or made out of synthetic fibre, will create the perfect environment for your genitals to grow Candida. And at the very least, can make sore skin even worse because of the tight, damp conditions. I'm not suggesting that you dress like a nun but as often as you can, wear a dress or skirt with bear legs. In the comfort of your home, wear nothing at all under your dress or skirt (doesn't that sound liberating!). And let the area breathe when you're sleeping too … meaning nothing under your night gown as well.

Sitting: Have you heard the news? "Sitting is the new smoking." I'm not going to get into the risks to the rest of your health if you sit for too long each day (because you can research that yourself); I am going to say that sitting on delicate and sore vulvar skin too much, isn't going to help anything. But I get it. Many of us have to sit for hours a day just to earn a living. (I've been thinking of making a new policy in my clinic where I set a timer on the computer and every 15 minutes we all get up and do a little on-the-spot dance for a minute!) The point is that you can work in breaks from all that sitting. Also consider getting a cushion for your sore *"down under"*. You may have to try a few out before you find the one that's just right for you (Goldilocks!). And if you're one of the keeners who bikes to work, or does a significant amount of biking, pay special attention to the bike seat too. You're working so hard to make this area comfortable, that you also need to consider sitting in a "pounds per square inch on your greater vaginal area" – type of way!

*FYI as I type this I am sitting on a cushion that I found at Bed Bath and Beyond. It's meant for a kitchen chair I think, but it works really well for me. If I go without it and type for longer than about 15 minutes, my labia gets sore, probably just because of less circulation getting to the area.

CHAPTER 6

Is Candida part of your Lichen Sclerosis picture?

I REMEMBER THE first time that I heard the word Candida. I thought: *How can something with the word "candy" in it be a bad thing?* Oh to be that innocent again! Up until then I'd had the occasional "yeast" infection diagnosis but (probably like many of you) I had no idea that the Y-e-a-s-t in Yeast Infection was part of a fungus family called Candida.

I was around 11 when I had my first "yeast" infection and my first exposure to anti-fungal vaginal creams like Canesten or Monistat. It's surprising actually, that it didn't happen sooner because I was a kid who took a lot of antibiotics. You know that campaign that they had a few years ago: Not All Bugs Need Drugs? Well I think they had the opposite one when I was growing up.

Antibiotics have been both a blessing and a curse on this planet. Certainly before their discovery and wide utilization of them, people died regularly of things like fevers and sore throats. There's no question that antibiotics have saved countless lives. But at what price? And have we become complacent with our personal health and maintenance preferring the convenience of swallowing a pill when something goes awry, to daily prevention?

Similar to the story of vaccinations, antibiotics really became mainstream at a time when the general living conditions for people vastly improved. Sanitation, fresh air and access to food year round are things that you and I take for granted in the 21st century but there was a time when living past the age of 30 was rare, largely because of living conditions.

So antibiotics were administered for nearly everything and people started living a lot longer in their better conditions. But was it the antibiotics or the change in living conditions that made people live longer?

Antibiotics are "anti" life. They destroy bacteria. The Germ Theory tells us that we are healthy unless we are invaded by bacteria (or fungus or viruses). Credited to Louis Pasteur, the Germ Theory survives today. But another theory (one that was not adopted by mainstream medicine yet has lingered, and has had numerous medical systems spring from it, only to be wiped out by the American Medical Association) is that we already have these bacteria, viruses and fungi in us (largely) and that they live harmoniously inside of us unless something (an "exciting factor") upsets the balance. This is called the Pleomorphic Theory and it was postulated by a contemporary of Louis Pasteur's named Antoine Béchamp. In fact on his death bed Pasteur was quoted as having said, "Béchamp was right".

My doctor explained the "Yeast infection" this way: *When you take antibiotics they kill the bacteria that caused your sore throat but they aren't very discriminating, also killing lots of other bacteria as well... even the good bacteria that you need. When those bacteria are wiped out, then the yeast is no longer in balance and grows out of control, to give you the symptoms of a Yeast Infection."* God bless the good doctor but his solution was another drug to kill the fungus.

Jeepers. It never occurred to me then but Béchamp's theory must be correct if we have Candida already in us. In this case the antibiotics were an "exciting factor" that killed the bacteria that keep Candida from multiplying out of control. Hmm, then not only do we always have Candida in our bodies but we also have "good" bacteria that keep the Candida in balance!!

I remember hearing my mom tell the story of how I ended up in the emergency room every month from the time that I was 18 months old to 3 years old, because of tonsillitis. So every month for a year and a half I was given MORE "good" bacteria destroying antibiotics! Sheesh! Didn't it occur to anyone to ask why this kept happening? And wouldn't it be nice if that was the end of my antibiotic story. But it was not. I took them a lot... eventually developing pretty severe symptoms from simple penicillin and then from sulpha drugs.

Recent research tells us that those "good" bacteria that are being wiped out by drugs like antibiotics and steroids (not to mention GMO foods), are a HUGE part of our immune systems. It turns out that once the brain has developed in the womb, then the very same material is used to create the stomach. All of those "good" bacteria are necessary for proper communication between the brain, the gut and the spinal cord. It's like we have another brain right in our bellies! (Actually Samuel Hahnemann knew this over 300 years ago! He called it the Gemut or "Body mind".)

Alright so now that you have a bit of understanding about your bacteria and how it gets out of balance and grows too many pathogenic and opportunistic organisms like Candida, you may have an idea why this yeast can be part of the Lichen Sclerosis picture. Remember in my story that I kept getting sick and being given more antibiotics and then I was given antifungals? What the medical system doesn't want to acknowledge is that "anti" medicines do not heal. This is the Law of Opposites (treat the problem with its opposite). It can suppress symptoms for a time and make you feel better but it does not heal the original problem, and it causes a lot more (problems) than you started with. And to top it off, your original problem can re-surface too!

In my case, the problem was likely that both of my parents smoked and I was really sensitive to cigarette smoke. Back then no one realized that exposing your kids to second hand smoke was potentially harmful! And my parents wouldn't listen to my protests about smoking in the car, which may have been another reason that I got so many throat infections (victim). So my body responded to these "exciting factors" by creating an inflammation in my throat. And it made me miserable so my parents took me to the doctor and antibiotics were given. The original problem (the cigarette smoke) was not dealt with and now a bunch of my immune system was knocked out. Then the little girl I was playing with next door came down with Strep throat and because my immune system was down from the antibiotics AND the cigarette smoke exposure, I got sick too. And just when I'd gotten through that, I fell off the back of dad's truck and the ER doc diagnosed Scarlett Fever! You guessed it, more antibiotics… and so it goes until finally my poor vagina was over-run by Candida and needed something to kill the fungus.

Do you see? The original problem(s) were never dealt with, only suppressed with more (and more!) drugs. So after several rounds of anti-fungal creams, which I eventually started having allergic reactions to, I needed topical steroids to suppress the symptoms from my immune system not being able to keep "bad" bugs in check. (And if you read chapter 2, then you know the problems that the topical steroids can cause to skin.)

But no one sat me down and said: *Hey, maybe you need to look at cleaning up what you're eating and consider taking a probiotic and maybe some Caprilic acid.* That information didn't come until much later and (sadly) not from a medical doctor.

So consider this chapter to be me sitting you down and saying… Maybe Candida is part of your LS picture and if so, here are some things you can do right now, to get you on the road to recovery! (And by the way, antibiotics can be life savers but save them for a true "life or death" situation because the time of *The End of Antibiotics* on this planet is quickly approaching due to over-prescribing and because they've been routinely fed to animals that we eat every, single day.)

How would you know if Candida is part of your picture? Do you suffer from...?

- Vaginal yeast infections (itching, burning, vaginal discharge, pain during sex, soreness and even a rash in the area)
- Thrush (yeast infection in your mouth)
- Brain fog/poor concentration
- Food & chemical sensitivities
- Problems with depression and/or anxiety
- Irregular bowels and/or IBS symptoms/chronic flatulence
- Headaches
- Extreme fatigue/lethargy
- Dry mouth/white coated tongue/bad breath
- Poor libido
- Rectal itching

This is not a complete list but you get the idea.

There are probably hundreds of books that can give you a super-rigid approach to eating to kill Candida. So if you are really drawn in that direction, then go ahead and check some of them out.

I am not a fan of being THAT rigid however, for two reasons...

1. If you've got LS, you're already suffering! Chronic itchy/irritated skin in your genitals is super-stressful! And as we've learned, is already taxing your Adrenal glands and adding to inflammation. So a really rigid diet is going to stress you out even further and it'll likely put you into a "victim" state-of-mind which (hello!) your vagina is already expressing.
2. There is a school of thought that says if you deny Candida a food supply, it will actually grow larger and expand its tentacles further in an attempt to feed itself. That doesn't sound like a good gamble to me!

Later in the book, I'm going to get into what to eat in order to heal/avoid LS but for now specific to Candida, I recommend the following:

Get on a Homeopathic dose of Candida (see chapter 4)

Blood Type Eating: Find out your blood type and follow the basic guidelines for that type. Why? Because your blood type will help to determine which foods your immune system considers "friend" or "foe". And the ones that are not considered friends will be attacked. What does an "attack" look like? You guessed it… inflammation. So you want to do everything that you can to calm down your immune response and make sure it is nice and healthy to attack things that really aren't good for you, instead of foods you eat on a daily basis. Your doctor may have a record of your blood type, but likely not. Check to see if he or she will order one for you and what the cost will be. OR you can order DIY kits on-line (www.4yourtype.com/original-home-blood-typing-kit) *FYI chapter 7 gives you more information on blood type eating and provides a basic list of foods for each type.

Fermented Foods and/or Probiotics: You'll want to incorporate fermented foods into your daily eating. This is a really key part of your recovery because these foods will help to re-seed your garden! In other words this is where you're going to get the "good" bacteria to put back into your body. Why fermented foods instead of a probiotic supplement? I have nothing against a good supplement (I love Renew Life's probiotics and Dr. Mercola's) but get this… a serving of fermented vegetables will have more bacteria in it than your whole bottle of probiotics! Now maybe there are some new ones that have come out since I read that statistic, but the point is that eating bacteria in your food is a much more cost effective way of re-populating your "good" bacteria and healing your body. Plus, by varying your fermented fair, you'll be exposing yourself to different strains.

Some examples of fermented foods: sauerkraut; kimchi; organic kefir; organic, plain yogurt with active bacteria; pickles (without vinegar) and kambucha.

**Here's the rule: DO NOT PURCHASE ANY FERMENTED FOODS FROM THE SHELF. They MUST be in the refrigerator and labeled "Raw"! If not, they will not have any of the bacteria left because it will have been destroyed by making them shelf-stable. Or make your own. (I hear it's pretty simple, if you're that type, which I'm really not…)

For those of you who don't know what kambucha is, it's fermented tea. Again, do not purchase any that is on the shelf or in a can. It should be in a bottle and it will have "stuff" on the bottom which is the glorious bacteria that your body needs! Don't be frightened though, it's pretty darn tasty… even reminiscent of soda… and on that note, don't shake it before opening, just gently circle it.

My recommendation is to go slow with these kinds of foods. Otherwise you can get "die off" symptoms. You'll know them if you get them: belching, bloating, noise in your gut, flatulence; diarrhea. Start with a teaspoon daily and eventually work up to a teaspoon with each meal. Then you can increase to a tablespoon and maybe a ¼ cup of kefir or kambucha. (If you do find that you get "die off" symptoms even by going slow, then you may need to get a bottle of probiotics and use that for a few months, BEFORE being able to handle the fermented foods. Additionally taking a good digestive enzyme supplement is a good idea for overall health, and to help heal your wonderful gut.)

By the way kefir is a better choice than yogurt because the bacteria are added to the kefir AFTER it's been pasteurized. This means that you'll get a lot more bacteria in there than in any yogurt that you buy from the store because pasteurization destroys all bacteria, not just the "bad" guys.

Crude Candida Killers: You'll definitely want to employ some
herbal help to get the population of Candida back down to a manageable level. Some well-known Candida destroyers include: Oregano oil; Olive leaf extract; Pau d'arco; Garlic; Neem; Black Walnut; Apple cider vinegar; Caprylic acid;

Coconut oil and Garlic.   If you go to a reputable health food store, they'll likely have some great formulations for Candida.   I am really grateful for New Roots and their combo called: Candida Stop (Black walnut; Garlic; Pau d'arco; Selenium, Echinacea root, Oregano; 3 types of Caprylic acid; Suma root and Grapefruit seed extract).   It's a good idea to employ a number of these herbs at the same time, in case the Candida learn to fight against just one or two that you might be taking for a while.   Conversely, if you're on one product (like the New Roots one above) for some time, change to a different combo with different ingredients after three months.

You can also learn to eat more coconut oil.   I love melting it in my coffee each morning.   And throughout the day you can enjoy it in herbal tea too, and you can cook with it - as long as you're okay with the slight change of flavor that it brings to your foods.   Not only is coconut oil excellent for your health because of its medium chain triglycerides (good fat!) but it's also an anti-fungal because it has caprylic acid in it.   And feel free to slather it on your body... you'll even get some of the nutritional benefits *that* way!

Acid or Alkaline? This is a controversial topic because those in the natural health field insist that our bodies are generally too acidic and need to be more alkaline, while those in the scientific community like to de-bunk the whole idea saying that your body will naturally turn all that you put into it, to the correct PH or it couldn't survive.   My understanding is that both are correct.   But I think there is a difference between merely surviving and THRIVING.   (And my simplistic understanding is that your body keeps the blood in a narrow range for life and ergo the kidneys will respond by either being more alkaline or more acidic, but that the saliva will vary greatly depending on your diet.)

But back to the surviving or thriving idea... isn't it interesting that Candida can't grow in an alkaline body?   (You may also be interested to know that cancer can't either.)   This is because these types of cells thrive in anaerobic environments.   In other words, they can't live in oxygen!   So if the cells of your body are healthy and oxygenated by the way that you take care of yourself, you won't be able to grow Candida any longer.

An easy way to get your body Alkaline (that is, in a state that doesn't support the life of Candida) is by using Barley greens. You can likely find some at your local health food store but the ones that I took are: **Barley Power by Green Supreme** (www.greensupreme.net). I took about 20 daily (they aren't very big and I stretched them through the day) along with my other Candida measures, and I felt I no longer suffered with Candida symptoms at about week three. As a side benefit, these have over 3,000 enzymes in them, so you can skip taking an additional digestive enzyme if you choose them.

*But please don't think that you can just take these and not put any attention into how you are feeding your beautiful body. It's like building a house... you need a good, strong foundation to build on. And you can't get that simply by swallowing a bunch of supplements.

Flower Essences: And finally, consider taking Australian Bush Flower Essences Green Essence combo (ausflowers.com.au). Flower Essences are similar to Homeopathic remedies because they are "vibrational" or "energy" medicine but be clear, they are not Homeopathic remedies. What the Green Essence bottle says is: "a vibrational infusion of traditional green herbs."

This particular Essence combo is really helpful for working with Candida. In and of themselves Flower Essences won't cure an actual disease, but they will help in conjunction with Homeopathic treatment and lifestyle changes, and they will make it easier for the sufferer to see some of their beliefs and patterns, which will help them to resolve the underlying reason(s) for their disease.

In the case of Candida it is an opportunistic organism so the sufferer generally has some sort of "victim" state that can be palliated by the use of this essence combo, while other action is taken to deal with the Candida. Additionally, Flower Essences make it easier to take better care of you. You know how when you feel miserable (like after a break-up!) you don't want to get up in the morning or eat and maybe you just sit around and drink wine or eat ice cream? Well Flower Essences somehow manage to help short-circuit that kind of response. So by taking this combo when targeting specific lifestyle changes to heal the condition of Candida overgrowth, it will make it much easier to stick with my other suggestions.

> *Could you and your partner be sharing a "yeast infection"? It's possible that you could be re-infecting each other. While a treatment of anti-fungal cream for his "package" could help, I love Tamanu oil because it is non-chemical and actually good for your skin plus it is a great anti-fungal topical treatment (look for it at your local health food store). You can use it too... rub liberally around affected area and use your finger to insert some into your vagina until yeast symptoms are gone. Additionally, get your partner to follow the same eating that you are. You'll both be a lot healthier!*

CHAPTER 7

The LS Healing "Diet" (Nope, this isn't the one that tells you what you should and shouldn't eat but hang in there cause it's coming!)

MANY YEARS AGO I read a book by Sondra Ray entitled: The Only Diet There Is. I loved her approach because essentially she said that the only diet anyone should follow is one that severely restricts negative thinking. And then she went on to give a month's worth of daily affirmations to say in front of a mirror. Sound advice! (Ha-ha pun intended.)

I was reminded of Ms. Ray's wisdom in preparing to write this chapter because it is similar. What I'm about to tell you may sound quite radical. But here goes: I want you, my dear reader (and LS sufferer) to consider putting yourself on a Sex fast... The Fast Sex Diet if you will (and here the word "fast" means *to abstain from* NOT *at lightning speed!*).

This was part of my recovery. In fact, it was part of the entire spiritual experience/miracle that I had. I was directed (remember the monk who called me at the beginning of the book?) to not have intercourse and not to give oral sex for several months.

I can hear your objections from here... "Oh my god my boyfriend would NEVER be okay with that!" "What IS she thinking?!" "Okay now I want my money back for this stupid book!"

This chapter is written from a traditional male/female interaction because that was my experience. I intend no exclusion or disrespect to other sexual orientations. If you are in a lesbian relationship, only you will know if your sexual activity contributes to your LS suffering or not but please finish the chapter even if it doesn't seem to, so that you can consider some of the deeper aspects of sexual activity as it relates to the condition of Lichen Sclerosis.

But let's explore this radical concept a bit. Consider ... if you came to see me with a chronic sore thumb because you kept hitting it with a hammer, I'd advise you to stop hitting it as much as possible. Additionally I'd give you Homeopathic remedies to heal the thumb AND the underlying reason why you keep hitting yourself with a hammer (in the first place). Plus I'd recommend dietary changes and supplements that would help with the inflammation – not *that* much different from if you came to see me with Lichen Sclerosis!

Do you get the analogy... every time you have sex, you are causing damage to the area, just like you would be by hammering your thumb over and over again. And the fact that you choose to have sex, in spite of the consequences to an already sore area, is likely a large part of the underlying reason for the LS.

In the case of Lichen Sclerosis the damage from continued sexual activity is two-fold, because you know that having sex generally makes things worse, but (if you're like I was) you can't imagine holding out on your partner like that. As women, we've been trained from birth to be care-givers and somewhere sex becomes part of that.

So by saying: *Honey I'm sorry but I've got this problem and whenever we're intimate it gets worse for a few days, so I need to not do it for a while. Can you support me in this and know that I love you, and that it's nothing personal?*

We feel guilty and like we aren't performing our duty to our partner. Or maybe you don't even feel free to voice your wants and needs this way to your partner. In that case every time that you have sex, even though you suffer for it afterwards (or maybe even during), you are creating a "victim" disease state. Whether it's victim, or guilt and shame for even considering asking for what you need, all of those feelings are contributing to the entire cycle of LS suffering.

For me, the guilt and the victim were completely relieved by my signing on for a wild spiritual journey that had rules about what I could and could not do sexually. This was just what I needed (the universe really does always provide!) because I had never felt that I had that power before. Now, it wasn't *me* saying I couldn't do it, it was a commitment I had made to a process greater than myself. (So if that's something that you need ladies, here you go… *"I'm sorry honey, but my Homeopathic physician says that I can't have sex for (like) 3 months, so that I can take the time that I need to heal down there."*)

It was a huge blessing to have the "burden" of sex taken off the table. Don't get me wrong, I enjoyed sex with my partner very much. But I never felt like I was the one initiating it or that I had the option to say "no" without being shamed for it (and honestly, I may have been the one doing all the shaming!). And in those moments, physical pain and suffering were a lot less painful than the shame and guilt that I felt.

Understand that I'm not suggesting that you give up physical pleasure but perhaps that you abstain from intercourse and giving oral sex, as I did. I was told that it was part of preparing me for what was to come spiritually, and I accepted that. But it really opened up a whole new world of learning about how to pleasure myself and also to being completely open to having my partner do that for me, without any expected reciprocation. I think there is a huge spiritual lesson here about the Sacred Feminine and how female pleasure is part of the health of the world. I was doing a lot of meditating at that time and honestly, sometimes the experiences that I had in meditation and in sexual pleasure were indistinguishable. And both helped me to relax and be a much nicer person to be around! Best of all, my greater vaginal area healed.

Receiving only, was hard to learn because I'm a giver, and likely you are too. The idea of only receiving pleasure was just wrong. Haven't we been taught this since we were toddlers? As a society we do this all the time... we give our little ones something and then if they don't think to share it, we shame them for it! I think the fine line between raising a child and breaking their spirit is super-blurry. Seriously, parenting is THE hardest job. And then we grow up and the only time that we get pure-unadulterated-just-for-me pleasure is when we pay someone to give it to us in the form of a massage or a spa day or a fine meal with desert & wine. And what do we call it? "My *guilty* pleasure!"

So my recommendation is 3 months away from intercourse. And for the sake of helping you to learn how to receive (only), make it about giving oral sex as well. However you may "give" in other ways but only if you REALLY want to. Your partner can (and is strongly encouraged to) give you pleasure however you would like. And you are encouraged to make love to yourself as often as you wish and however you wish, as long as you don't cause pain or injury. (As a side note, you and your partner may wish to learn about the OM (Orgasmic Meditation) which is where a partner gives pleasure by stroking the clitoris a certain way for 12 minutes, with no expectation of reciprocation.)

Think of it this way: The diamond industry has convinced us that if a man really wants to marry that special someone, then he should spend 3 months of his salary on an engagement ring. So in comparison, these 3 months are a bargain! (Of course it goes without saying that if you are not healed in 3 months, you can continue the diet for longer.) And by the way, this will be a real journey for your partner. Likely he will learn and grow from it, and your sex life will become better than ever as he understands (perhaps for the first time) about the sacred spirituality of sex with a woman. *And it would be an excellent time for him to read chapter 14 of Naomi Wolf's book: Vagina (see chapter 1).*

Not having sex was part of my LS healing journey so I know this is an integral part of yours. And you probably know it too, by the level of discomfort you're feeling with considering it. But please do. Toss aside the notion that it is better to give than to receive and do GIVE yourself pleasure and RECEIVE pleasure from your partner without HAVING to give any back, unless your heart is singing that it wants to. I know this concept is likely really abstract right now, as you read about it, but removing all the sexual "have to's" will liberate so many of the false beliefs that are contributing to your Lichen Sclerosis condition. You will be taking a giant step toward living your authentic life!

But please, please, please don't just make this about abstaining, because that is definitely NOT the point. The point is your **pleasure** and **choice**. Simply not having any sexual activity will be like a punishment and may not get you any closer to healing LS. Oh your skin may heal because of inactivity, but likely your symptoms will return once you resume your sex life. And if your partner simply will not support the work in this chapter, then you need to consider if this is someone who is indeed worthy of you. Because my friend, you are definitely worth the Fast Sex Diet!

CHAPTER 8

What should you eat/avoid for healing LS?

CONGRATULATIONS! YOU'VE COME so far, and I'm willing to bet that you're feeling a lot better. For many of you, this chapter will be a piece of cake (well, one made with almond or coconut flour only!). But for some of you, it may be where you meet your greatest resistance to healing Lichen Sclerosis. Here's a list of common reasons why we are attached to our food choices:

a) We find them comforting
b) They are convenient
c) We believe they are the way to maintain health and avoid cardiovascular disease
d) We don't want to be that "weirdo" in the family who eats differently from everyone else *(Hello Uncle Waldo! I do notice you glaring at me!!)*
e) We are morally/ethically opposed to eating certain foods
f) All of the above!

I get it. I run into these resistances every day in my Homeopathic practice. But remember in the last chapter when we talked about hitting your thumb daily with a hammer? Well our food choices can be the same as assaulting your body with a hammer (or worse). Why? Because most of the foods we eat cause inflammation and LS is an inflammatory condition. So no treatment plan for Lichen Sclerosis could be complete without helping you navigate the myriad of food choices and misinformation, so that you can create the healthiest regimen for your long term health and vitality, as well as relief of your Lichen Sclerosis symptoms.

Eating = Inflammation? Remember what you learned at the beginning of chapter 3 about inflammation being the body "attacking"? Well in the case of eating, many of the foods most of us eat will trigger your immune system to start attacking them. Just think about the damage a war can do... all that destruction. It's no different inside of you. If your immune system is attacking the food that you eat while your gastro intestinal system is attempting to digest it, that entire system will be attacked too! And that means that there will be tiny holes where there should NOT be holes. This sets off a vicious cycle because food particles that otherwise might not be a problem, can fall through those holes and now your immune system will attack them simply because they are in an area of the body where they're not supposed to be. And to make matters worse, the part of your body where that foreign food happens to be when it gets attacked, will suffer collateral damage.

I can't emphasize this enough: **To really recover and live happily ever after *"down under"* you need to clean up your eating**. War is hell and if your body is constantly attacking food as well as undigested particles that slip through holes, it won't have the energy to take care of basic maintenance. Soon it'll start prioritizing what is and is not necessary for survival. Maintenance of skin integrity in the genital area will be placed at the bottom of the list!

Paleo/Primal eating: Essentially I do recommend (and follow) a "Paleo" type of approach. For those of you who aren't familiar with this food trend here is a cute definition that I just found on a quick Google search:

"The Paleo Diet is an effort to eat like we used to back in the day...WAY back in the day. If a caveman couldn't eat it, neither can you."

That's kind of it, in a nutshell. If it's been processed (and/or microwaved) it's not really "food" any longer because it will not feed your body. And instead of adding to your health, it will take from it and (you guessed it) cause inflammation in the process! Additionally, spend the extra money to ensure that you are eating the highest quality food possible. You may think organics are too expensive but if you can afford it, you are actually getting about 80%

more nutrition than in conventional foods. Plus the food won't have chemical additives that you don't want. The one exception is in seafood. Do not buy organic seafood because this automatically means that it has been farmed. Farmed seafood is toxic and it is causing a lot of problems for our oceans. Do your research and then just say "no" to farmed fish!

By the way, cavemen didn't have access to soda pop, fruit juice or alcohol. Many of my patients are shocked to hear that the only beverage they need is water. And you do need water! Chronic dehydration could be part of your LS picture or it could be masquerading as other symptoms in your body. Divide your weight in pounds by 2 and then divide that number by 8 and you'll know how many 8oz cups of water you need daily in order to be healthy. But add more on days when you work out and/or sweat. And be sure that you use a clean and energetically "alive" source of water.

The key to this kind of eating, is avoiding grains and sugar. Though we were taught from very early on (remember health class in elementary school?) that grains are healthy, the evidence and research does not support that teaching. It turns out that grains, once eaten, rapidly turn to sugar in your body! And yes, I mean whole grains too. Read on…

Weston Price (www.westonaprice.org) was a dentist at the turn of the 20th century who travelled the world in search of the answer to the question: *Why are so many people suddenly showing up with dental cavities and crooked teeth in my office (especially young children)?* What he found was that our new "modern" diet was altering the structure of our faces (limiting the amount of room we had for teeth) and causing inflammation. He noted that traditional cultures that had never heard of appendicitis (or *inflammation* of the appendix), suddenly learned about it when their people changed over from traditional foods to the "Western" way of eating. As it turns out, cavities in the mouth are just one of the symptoms of a body that is besieged by inflammation.

Indeed anthropological digs show that before we became an Agrarian culture (growing our own food), there was no death from inflammatory conditions such as diabetes, heart disease or cancer. And yes, there are those who argue that we simply didn't live long enough (because of starvation or predators) to die from inflammation back then. While that may have some merit, short life span is no longer a concern for humans. Now we can learn from the past *and* make our advances work *for* us, not against us!

Most of us were never taught that grains turn to sugar in your body. But they do. Savvy food companies have switched to "whole" grains now in an attempt to sway us back to our love affair with grains, but largely whole grains will also quickly turn to sugar after you eat them. They are simply too processed – meaning they aren't at all what nature intended and they lack vital nutrients.

So let's think about that for a minute … if you eat a bowl of oatmeal, and it turns to sugar, that's a **whole lot** of sugar! You'd never eat THAT much sugar!! Who knew? And who doesn't add something to sweeten that oatmeal, plus milk? Did you know that cow's milk has sugar in it? It's called Lactose, and a cup of milk (all milk, even skim) has 16 grams of carbohydrate (that turns to sugar) in it. When you think of it this way, you can begin to see how that bowl of oatmeal just stopped being a "health" food, right?

Some would argue that steal cut oats are good for you. And I would say that **IF** you do not suffer from a debilitating condition like Lichen Sclerosis, and **IF** you have normal blood pressure, normal triglycerides, normal blood glucose and normal fasting insulin numbers then yes, you could handle a serving of gluten free steal cut oats a couple of times a week. Why Steal cut? Because the oats have been minimally processed meaning that there is a lot more nutrition in these oats (that will assist your body in assimilating them) in addition to a certain type of fibre (called: resistant) that will not quickly raise your blood sugar (and cause an insulin spike/inflammation) but will keep it level for several hours. The downside is that steal cut oats take longer to make, so they are not convenient.

That is the other key to this kind of eating... you need to be committed to spending a bit of time thinking about and preparing your food. Real food takes some prep time. But honestly, once you get the hang of it, it's not difficult. I can make myself a healthy meal of steamed or sautéed vegetables and scrambled eggs with onions in them, plus some coconut yogurt with (previously frozen) mixed berries for desert, in about 15 minutes!

A word about wheat: Hopefully you are taking this chapter very seriously and have already decided to stop eating grains. Good for you! And you know that wheat is a grain so it's gone. (Yay!)

But here's the thing... many people come back for their follow up appointment and say to me: "I've mostly stopped the wheat. I'll only have a piece of toast twice a week or I allow the odd bit of croutons when I'm dining out." Believe it or not, "them's fight'n words" to your immune system. Size doesn't matter here! A virus is so small that you can't even see it with your eyes but if you are exposed to it, it can make you sick for several weeks or longer (depending on the virus). Well you *can* see those croutons and you *can* see that toast just fine, so imagine what that much wheat can do to your immune system.

I'm mentioning this because, of all the grains, wheat likely causes the most damage to your immune system. (For more information about this consider reading *Wheat Belly* by William Davis, MD and *Grain Brain* by David Perlmutter, MD.) As the story goes, wheat was changed on our little planet back in 1960. It isn't that it was genetically modified but hybridized (meaning they combined genetically different strains of wheat until they came up with the "modern" wheat of today). It is said that this wheat will stand up to strong winds better, but it also has a lot more gluten in it than the wheat that our ancestors ate. (Gluten is a protein that gives wheat its "gluey" texture, and it's what people are reacting to when they have Celiac disease.) Additionally if it isn't 100% certified organic wheat (and it almost never is when you're eating out) it will have large amounts of Glyphosate in it. Glyphosate is a chemical herbicide that has not only been labeled as a "probable carcinogen" (cancer causing) in humans, but its job is to destroy weeds. What are weeds but plants that are growing in the wrong place at the wrong time? One man's weed is another man's... you get the idea. But my point is that Glyphosate also destroys the villi (finger-like structures that allow absorption of nutrients) in your intestines. You really need your villi (not to mention your "good-guy" bacteria which this herbicide also kills) in order to be healthy!! Monsanto (the company that makes Glyphosate/Roundup) claims that the dose of Glyphosate that we are exposed to in food isn't enough to harm us, but can they really make that claim with any level of certainty? (Besides often big companies will claim that their studies prove efficacy and safety but it takes an independent study - one done by no one with a *financial interest* in showing safety - to expose the truth.)

And here's a "fun" fact... By spraying the plants again just before harvest (called "dessicating") it will dry them, cause them to produce extra seeds, and help to get a jump start on next year's weeds (2013 Journal Entropy – Dr. Stephanie Seneff on Celiac and Glyphosate use.) **This practice means that you and I are being exposed to a lot more glyphosate than was ever studied for safety.** It's interesting to note that Celiac disease has exploded in the past 15 years – since dessicating and GMO crops have come on the scene. (As mentioned in chapter 3, sulphur can be considered for helping your gut (therefore your entire body!) to heal from Glyphosate exposure in your food.)

Glyphosate and even gluten aside, this new wheat is completely foreign to your body. And you (now) know what your body likes to do with foreign invaders. Clinically wheat consumption has been linked to a myriad of health conditions including Alzheimer's disease, Migraines, Diabetes, Colon cancer, Arthritis, Vitiligo, Hair loss and Acne (to name a few). And it can give you a big belly! So in case you were on the fence about whether or not to be really religious about going wheat free, this list (and your LS symptoms) should convince you :O)

A word about the "F" word (Fat): This innocent nutrient has become the catalyst for many arguments regarding healthy eating. It was demonized years ago because of a faulty theory called "The Lipid Hypothesis". (For more information about this consider reading *The Great Cholesterol Myth* by Jonny Bowden, PH.D., C.N.S. and Stephen Sinatra, M.D., F.A.C.C. or *GOOD Calories, BAD Calories* by Gary Taubes)

Certainly there are bad fats, but they're probably not what you think. A good rule of thumb is that anything that is in a package that you couldn't open up in the middle of one of those super-quiet moments at the Symphony (cause it would make a **big/crinkling** noise!), is going to have bad fat in it. In other words, eat *real* food and you'll avoid *bad* fat. It's that simple.

Let's think about those cavemen again... they wouldn't be exposed to packaged foods with fats that had to be processed in order to be shelf stable. But they *were* eating animal fats, yet they were lean/mean/hunting machines, free of inflammatory illness! The idea that animal fats are bad for us has been discredited. Yes, eating it will raise your cholesterol, but studies prove that sick people with the lowest cholesterol levels will die sooner than those who have high cholesterol. Maybe because when we don't eat fat, we can't metabolize a whole bunch of nutrients in our diet that are fat soluble. And, my dear LS sister, we need our cholesterol if for no other reason, than to moisturize and lubricate our skin!! (But there are a lot of reasons besides that.)

Eating fat as nature intended is anti-inflammatory and it will help you to lose weight AND have a healthy heart. Plus, it's what will keep you satiated now that you won't be eating grains. Fat makes you full and keeps you full for a lot longer than grains ever could – all without raising your blood sugar! Incidentally it's sugar and grains that will raise your triglycerides – which is the measurement for fat in your blood. Kind of makes you wonder why we ever believed that Lipid Hypothesis in the first place, doesn't it?

Just in case the "F" word has been out of your vocabulary for so long that you don't have a clue what foods I'm talking about, here's a list to get you started: avocado; chia; coconuts, coconut oil; flax seeds, flax oil; olives, olive oil; (organic, grass fed and ideally raw) butter, cream, yogurt, cheese; (organic, grass-fed) meats; wild salmon, halibut, sardines; (organic and/or raw) walnuts, pecans, macadamia nuts; (organic or raw) dark chocolate.

Notice that: margarine, corn oil, canola oil and that vegetable-alternative-to-lard are not on the list. Just think of how much effort and technology are needed to make canola and corn into oil or to make the completely "man-made" butter-like product called margarine. Cavemen definitely wouldn't have eaten any of these *bad* fats and neither should you.

Breakfast ideas: Many people find breakfasts to be the most challenging part of this kind of eating so I recommend that you go to your favorite search engine and type in: *Paleo breakfasts*. Additionally pick up a couple of Paleo recipe books that feel right for you (so you can also find desert ideas too!). But here's an easy rule: the more you can make breakfast look like last night's dinner, the more on track you'll be!

Here are a couple of my favorite breakfasts:

Breakfast pudding:
1 Avocado (peeled and cut into 1 inch pieces)
Coconut milk to cover
2 Tsp. ground chia seeds (color does not matter)
2 Tsp. raw cacao powder
1 Handful of fresh or frozen spinach or kale
½ - ¾ Cup of berries (mixed usually and previously frozen)
6-8 Cashews or other nut(s) or a handful of seeds (like raw pumpkin)
½ Serving of pea protein powder (use more if you wish but I do not enjoy the taste)
Stevia to taste (I prefer liquid and generally use English toffee flavor – 30 drops; alter powdered stevia accordingly as you will need very little)
3 Shakes of Himalayan salt

Combine all ingredients in food processor or Magic Bullet, mix and enjoy!

Chia porridge:
3 – 4 Tbsp of ground chia seeds
¾ - 1 Cup of coconut milk
8 Drops of stevia
1 Tsp (or more) of coconut oil (added after cooking)
Combine ingredients with a whisk, bake in toaster oven at 350F for 6 minutes, mix in oil and enjoy. Once it's cooked it is very similar to cream of wheat. Add a boiled egg (to the meal) or a piece of last night's meat and some leftover veggies from dinner and you're set!

"Fruit" salad:
1 Handful of cherry tomatoes cut in half
1 Handful of cucumbers (skin removed if waxy) cut into bite-size pieces
A small amount of onion cut into tiny pieces for flavor
1/8 – ¼ Avocado cut into tiny pieces
Olive oil to coat everything (make sure it's organic and cold pressed and only purchase a small bottle so it won't go rancid before you finish it – 6 weeks max)
Himalayan salt, Herbamare seasoning and garlic powder – season with all, mixing and tasting until it is to your liking
Again you'll want to add a protein to this meal (egg, chicken, fish, steak, etc.)

There are plenty of grain-free recipes that you can use to make muffins and cookies (using almond flour and/or coconut flour, etc.) or even dinner rolls, to have on hand to add to your meals. If you feel you don't have the time to bake, consider hiring someone to do it for you, or barter with someone. In my practice, I have a couple of ladies who make extra money by baking for other patients who don't have the time but have the money.

A *sweet* thought: Many paleo eating plans include honey and maple syrup. I do not include much of either in my daily regimen because they will raise blood sugar. Yes, they are healthier sweeteners, and they each have a lot of nutrition that helps your body to process the sugar in them, but that doesn't mean that we should consume them all day, every day. Remember those cavemen… they were lucky to find a treat of some honey! So reserve these treats for special occasions only, and you'll do well to avoid them entirely (for a time) if you are dealing with Candida. FYI liquid Stevia is my go-to sweetener. It won't raise your blood sugar and it's made from a non-toxic plant that is 300 times sweeter than sugar. I tell folks to add only one drop at a time and taste it before adding more, cause (apparently) there really can be too much of a good thing!

***Paleo eating includes dairy. I have recommended that Lichen Sclerosis sufferers omit dairy from their diet because it may be part of the pathology. How? Mother Nature designed cow's milk with lots of naturally occurring hormones in it that tell a calf's body how to get big quickly. Consequently many human immune systems react to those cow hormones.

When I stopped eating dairy I didn't notice anything initially. And that's pretty common until you eat some of the food in question. For me it was accidentally eating a bit of ice cream a couple of weeks later. The next day my labia was really swollen and felt like I'd been punched. Seriously. I couldn't believe it! Often we don't realize how good we feel, until we (well) don't anymore. That's called perspective! And it was enough for me to swear off of dairy. Well that's not 100% accurate. I have my favorite Indian restaurant where I'll order Butter Chicken and as long as I don't actually eat the sauce, but only the chicken covered in it, I don't get a flare. So my immune system can handle a bit, and I know my limits.

You won't know if dairy is playing a part in your LS picture, until you omit it and then try it again (yes, that does include that little bit of cream in your coffee! FYI Cashew Milk is a pretty close second). 3 weeks of absti-nence is considered the gold standard for this sort of em-pirical testing.

Blood Type Eating: Dr. Peter J. D'Adamo brings us blood type eating in his book: *Eat Right 4 Your Type*. This is sound nutritional advice and part of what I teach all of my patients, not just my LS ones. The reason is that different blood types evolved at different rates on this planet and we are largely still suited to eat the same way that our original ancestors did. I've provided a really simplified version of what each of the blood types can eat and should avoid. Once you've confirmed your blood type, simply look at your list and modify your paleo eating to fit with your blood type. (Note: If your blood type recommendations conflict with paleo eating, go with the paleo. After all cavemen didn't have a clue what blood type they were!!) Why is this necessary? Because your particular blood type will identify certain foods as foreign and attack them, where someone else's type may not. You won't know how great you can feel until you try it!

Of course if you want to go more in depth in your blood type eating check out the book or go online (www.dada-mo.com). I understand there are even apps you can get now! But please don't make yourself crazy over this. The basics will do the trick, so maybe start there until you're looking for a new challenge in your life.

Be sure to listen to your body however. Hopefully this entire journey has helped you to honor your body's unique wisdom more and more, and feed-ing it is no exception. For example, when I gave birth to my second son I experienced a lot of complications and lost a lot of blood during the delivery and for a week afterward. Eventually I had to have an emergency surgery and by then I'd lost so much blood that my veins had collapsed and they had a heck of a time starting an IV. It took my body a long time to recover from that shock (I didn't have the Heilkunst healing system in my life yet!). I had been a vegetarian prior to that birth but couldn't do it for years after because I'd get to about week 3 of my menstrual cycle and CRAVE red meat like crazy. So I just gave in. I ate whatever meat that I felt like, when I felt like it until one day I literally heard a voice say: "You know, you don't need that meat anymore." That was shortly after the birth/blood loss trauma had been dealt with in my own Heilkunst healing journey. So I stopped eating it and there was no hardship whatsoever. That said, I am human just like you, and I ended up pushing myself too hard and burning the candle at both ends. I started displaying a cluster of symptoms that included anemia again. Eventually I realized that I had Hypothyroidism and Adrenal Fatigue (turns out the two conditions often go together). Part of my recovery included some certified organic, grass fed bison every couple of weeks, in addition to an iron supplement. What's super-interesting here is that I had identified (after I stopped the red meat) that it did trigger LS symptoms for me. They weren't the same as the milk… more itching and cracking of the skin but definitely noticeable. But this does NOT happen when I eat the bison. I don't have a scientific explanation but it does add to my great trust in the wisdom of my body. In case you haven't already figured it out, I am a blood type A – a natural vegetarian (though A's can have poultry and fish). I follow my blood type eating except for 2 occasions per month, and that's what works perfectly for me. So please, figure out what works perfectly for you, instead of just blindly doing what this book (or any other) tells you to.

A note about pork: I recommend that you avoid it. There must be a reason it's written into several of the world's major religions, right? The issue is that the DNA of "Porky" is too similar to your own. So if your Christmas ham has a virus or fungus attached to it, your immune system will not recognize it and you'll become infected with it. That means that while the meat may not fire up your immune system, the organism that it infected you with will. Samuel Hahnemann noted that some of his patients (way back in the 1700's!) never recovered, if they kept eating pork.

However I'll give you a loophole: If you purchase pork that has been raised correctly and fed correctly (certified organic, grass fed, SPCA certified, etc.), and if it has been cured traditionally and not with the use of carcinogenic chemicals, then (and only THEN) you can probably get away with a little bit on special occasions. For me a piece of bacon will cause a big LS flare! But I can eat several pieces (on special occasions) when I get the ones that meet all of the above criteria.

Blood Type O:

- **Emphasis: Red meats** (natural carnivore) and seafood (esp. if you are Asian/Eurasian ancestry)

However men past the age of 50 and women who are not menstruating should have iron/ferritin levels checked to make sure they do not get too high

- More often when stressed (as snacks)
- No more than 6 oz per meal – 1 serving per day is ideal
- Richly-oiled, cold water fish (eg. Cod, Herring, Mackerel – consume with strawberries to avoid over exposure to mercury)
- Best is grass-fed beef over grain fed
- O's have high stomach acid to digest meat

- **Eliminate dairy** (esp. if of African descent) (fermented dairy that is organic or raw and not made from skim milk may be ok if you've eliminated for 3 weeks and did not get a flare when re-introduced)
- Eggs limit to: 1 egg 4-5 times a week (none if African descent)
- Oils: best are monounsaturated (olive, flaxseed)
- Limit nuts & seeds (this fat can make O's gain weight)
- Beans & legumes in moderation
- **No grains**
- **Lots of vegetables**
- **Moderate fruit** (avoid super-sweet ones like tropical fruits; limit or avoid for Candida)
- Juices should be limited; vegetable over fruit but absolutely avoid apple and orange juices

Blood Type A:

- **Little Meat** – only some fish, poultry
- **Ideally vegetarian** (not vegan)
- Little fat and oils
- Nuts and seeds for protein (best are peanuts and pumpkins)
- Lots of beans and legumes (for protein)
- Lots of vegetables
- Grains ok for A (1 serving per day *but this conflicts with Paleo eating*) – limited wheat or **none is best**; need to balance wheat with alkaline foods (see fruits) to keep muscle tissue slightly alkaline (best for this type)
- **Little or no dairy**
- **Lots of fruit** – at least 3 times a day (limit or avoid for Candida); pineapple is excellent; start morning with small glass of warm water with juice of ½ fresh lemon (reduces mucus, stimulates digestion and elimination)
- Coffee/Alcohol: some red wine and coffee are beneficial as type A's tend to have low stomach acid (apple cider vinegar will work too)

Blood Type B:

- **Balanced** and wholesome diet, including dairy (moderation & organic only or raw and <u>not skim</u>; do the elimination for 3 weeks to be sure about this for you)
- If lactose intolerant – slowly incorporate, especially in fermented form
- Eat 3 square meals a day
- **Sensitive to wheat and gluten, and rye**
- Light, white meats (but **no chicken**) but also lamb, mutton, venison and rabbit (some beef)
- **Thrive on seafood**, especially deep-ocean fish (wild only! And eat with strawberries to avoid over exposure to mercury)
- Olive oil – 1 tablespoon a day

- No or few nuts and seeds – almonds, brazil, chestnuts, litchi, macadamia, pecans, walnuts are neutral so okay
- Few beans and legumes – kidney, lima, navy are best
- Grains – rice, spelt and (steel cut) oats are best... but limiting grains to only 1 serving or less is best *and this conflicts with Paleo eating*
- Lots of vegetables – avoid only artichokes, avocado, corn, olives, pumpkin, radishes, tomato
- **Lots of fruits (limit or avoid for Candida)** – avoid only coconuts (oil is okay though), pomegranates, rhubarb, star fruit, persimmons
- Avoid tempeh and tofu (soy)
- Spices: warming ones are best... ginger, horseradish, curry, cayenne pepper, parsley

Blood Type A/B:

*Most foods that are contraindicated for A types and B types are for AB too (some exceptions, such as tomatoes)

Some Challenges...

- Needs to eat protein (B), but has low stomach acid (A)
- Susceptible to low blood sugar
- Utilize calories best when tissue is alkaline
- Though less reactive to wheat gluten, wheat will still cause weight gain (and other problems as already discussed)

*Dairy good, like type B (make sure it is organic or raw, not skim; do the elimination for 3 weeks to be sure about this for you)

*Best protein - seafood and fish (eat with strawberries to avoid over exposure to mercury; avoid chicken (like type B)

*Eggs-good source of protein

*Can suffer from gall bladder problems

*Best fruits are more alkaline ones (grapes, plums & berries); worst fruits are mango, banana & guava; pineapples are excellent (for digestion); avoid oranges, but lemons are excellent

*Ideal to begin each day with a glass of warm water with freshly-squeezed juice of half a lemon to cleanse the system of mucus. Follow with diluted glass of grapefruit or papaya and then eat breakfast.

*Spices – sea salt and kelp; AVOID all pepper and vinegar; small amounts of sugar are allowed (not ideal) and chocolate (dark, organic or raw)

*Beverages - red wine, coffee (small amounts to promote stomach acid), green tea

*Breakfast – "Eat like a king" with protein!

Skim Milk: You may have noticed the recommendation to not drink skim milk. This is because skim milk is what farmers used to feed to the pigs and chickens. In other words it's garbage! When you remove the fat from milk 2 things happen…

1. No one wants to drink it or eat it because it's blue and because the texture is weird, so the milk producers add color and texture to entice you, AND…
2. Removing the fat exacerbates the carbs because no fat means there's nothing there to challenge how quickly all of those carbs turn to sugar in your body. Make no mistake: A "Skinny Latte'" is anything but.

Soy: I don't *do* soy. Did you know that if a baby is fed soy formula it is like giving her 3-4 birth control pills daily? That's because soy is estrogenic to the human body. This means that it will plug into the estrogen receptor cells in your body and behave like estrogen. Remember, we already have a whole lot of things in our environment that do this already. Even in Menopause, there are better ways to deal with uncomfortable symptoms than eating soy.

Additionally soy will fire up your immune system particularly in the area of your thyroid. That means that when your immune system attacks the soy, your poor thyroid will be attacked too and you could end up with Hypothyroidism… which makes you super-tired and can make you gain weight. Have I got your attention now?!

And if all that isn't enough, soy is an "excitotoxin" because it is naturally high in Glutamate. Glutamate can cause cancer, and it can also feed existing cancer cells. An excitotoxin is something that literally excites a cell to the point of death. (To learn about this and other "excitotoxins", go to www.russell-blaylockmd.com to read about Neurosurgeon Dr. Russel Blaylock's, research.) The take-home: Soy is not the health food that we've been led to believe it is.

Resistant Fibre Carbs: Right about now you might be wondering what you're going to use for fuel if you aren't eating grains and sugar. Well rest assured that eating vegetables, meat, fat and fruit will keep you going, as it did your ancestors! However I'd like to introduce you to a list of carbohydrate foods that I learned about from Dr. Alan Christianson, NMD in his book *The Adrenal Reset Diet* (www.theAdrenalresetdiet.com).

What's great about these carbs is that they often help people who have accumulated a lot of weight around their waist-lines, to lose it. This occurs because these foods provide a type of fibre (resistant - just like the steal cut oats) that does not cause a big spike in your blood sugar and also keeps you feeling satiated physically and emotionally for several hours. These resistant fibre foods can help your body to feel good, even if you are low in cortisol because of Adrenal Fatigue. (If you've been using topical steroid ointment for years, I'm talking to you!) Dr. Christianson explains that as cortisol levels drop naturally throughout the day, for some it'll become too low (causing sleep problems which lead to weight gain over time), so he has them increase the level of these types of carbs with each meal, to help balance the situation. If a large belly is your problem, this is one of the BEST solutions that I've seen so do check it out.

While Dr. Christianson and I agree on most things, I still recommend that my patients limit or avoid grains… especially when you are beginning your LS healing journey. Once you're feeling great, you can experiment with more grains on this list and see what happens.

Acorn squash, Adzuki beans, Banana (see below) Barley, Beets, Black beans, Blackberries, Blueberries, Brown rice, Butternut squash, Cannellini beans, Garbanzo beans (chickpeas), Grapefruit, Great northern beans, Hummus, Kidney beans, Kabocha squash, Lentils, Navy beans, Parsnips, Peas, Peach, Pinto beans, Potato (1/4c boiled only), Quinoa, Raspberries, Gluten free steal cut oats, Strawberries, Sweet potato, Turnips

Even ¼ of a small **banana that is still partly green**, is allowable a couple of times a week! (Can you tell I LOVE bananas?) *Limit or avoid if you are working on weight loss and/or Candida issue.

Potatoes should be cooked and refrigerated overnight BEFORE you eat them. That will change the starch.

Yum: Here's something that may surprise you… I encourage you to eat dark chocolate. There are sooo many health benefits linked to consumption of dark chocolate - from antioxidants and healthy fat, to feeding the good bacteria in your gut, to a natural anti-depressant! But it needs to be high quality. I always tell my patients, if it's going to pass through your lips, it had better be worthy! After all the point of this kind of eating is not deprivation, but finding healthy ways to feed your body (as well as your spirit).

The darker the chocolate, the healthier it'll be so go for at least 70% cacao and make sure it is organic at the least and raw is ideal. More and more natural food stores are carrying raw chocolate bars (I LOVE Zimt organic/raw/dairy free chocolate bars: www.zimtchocolates.com) and you can even find packages of chocolate covered almonds (for example) that use raw, dark chocolate. Also learn to read the nutrition label. If that chocolate bar has a bunch of carbs in it, then all that added sugar will impair chocolate's health promoting qualities. Look for something with a number of 13 or less carbohydrate per serving. It may take some time, but you will be able to re-train your taste buds not to need so much sweetness. Be sure to subtract the amount of fibre from the carbs to accurately know how many carbs are in there. Remember dark chocolate is so filling and satiating that you likely won't eat an entire serving, so that will lower the carb count too.

And when you're reading that nutrition label, note the kind of sugar/sweetener that is being used. Cane sugar and coconut sugar are ideal choices NOT High Fructose Corn Syrup or even Agave Nectar because they will impair your liver function and promote weight gain.

Do be cautious with chocolate however, if you are working on Candida issues and/or consider purchasing some of the newer chocolate bars that are sweetened only with a combination of Stevia and Erythritol but no sugar(s). (Some people may have digestive issues from Erythritol – a sugar alcohol that digests further down than maltitol, making it easier digested than maltitol, for many *but not all*.)

Agave nectar… yes or no? I think the bottom line is this: If you live somewhere where you can grow your own Agave and harvest the nectar yourself, in the proper way so that you consume it quickly and it doesn't have to go through a lot of processing, then likely it'll be a decent sugar substitute. Otherwise forget it because it is highly processed syrup. Sure it's low glycemic (meaning it doesn't cause a quick spike in blood sugar) but it does contribute to fatty liver disease and type 2 diabetes in the same way that High Fructose Corn Syrup Does. It isn't worth it.

**Consider taking a really good Digestive Enzyme supplement now. We are only born with so many (enzymes) and they get depleted by a standard North American Diet. Without digestive enzymes, you force your pancreas to work really hard and your body can "burn out" (and get sick) just trying to digest your cooked food. (Think about how tired you feel after a big, turkey dinner at Thanksgiving or Christmas!) Taking digestive enzymes and/or eating more raw foods means you'll have more energy and you'll be able to heal your gastro intestinal system a lot faster (meaning your LS will heal faster). Do make sure the supplement you choose has a good dose of Pancreatin in it and if you happen to be without your gallbladder, it's imperative that you include bile salts in your enzyme supplement.

CHAPTER 9

Supplements for healing LS

As a HEALTHCARE practitioner I like to think that I know a thing or 2 about nearly anything that has to do with keeping the body healthy, but you remember the old saying about hairdressers having the worst hair? Well I think at some point, I became a complacent know-it-all and simply forgot to apply some of the rules that I was teaching to my patients every day – to me! That's where these two ladies came to my rescue with their wonderful books!! Please consider reading them if you want to expand on your own knowledge of herbal and nutritional supplements...

1. *Eczema, Itchin' For A Cure* by Suzy Cohen (www.suzycohen.com) (I've mentioned Suzy a few times already.)
2. *The Forbidden Truth about Vitamins What You Don't Know Will Hurt You* by (Fellow Heilkunst physician!) Aleksandra Mikic, DHHP, DVHH, DPH (http://Shininghealth.net/)

What follows is a list of what I took as part of my Lichen Sclerosis healing protocol... (Unless mentioned, follow the directions on the label and/or consult with a health care provider.)

A good Multi-vitamin/mineral supplement: As inconvenient as it may be, the days of getting all of your nutritional needs met by the foods that you eat are gone. We've discussed many of the problems with our modern food supply already but additionally there's the very real problem of nutrient depletion from the soil. This happens in Organic farming as well as Industrial Agriculture. Not only are vitamins and minerals

disappearing at an alarming rate, but the "good" bacterium in our soil is too. Educate yourself; tell others and take your multi as an insurance policy.

That said, not just any Multi that you pick up at a big box store will do. Believe it or not, taking a low-quality vitamin supplement will be worse to your body than taking nothing at all! Isn't that amazing? There are a few reasons for this, but a major one is that nature intended for vitamins to be in a full complex. But for years vitamin manufacturers have synthesized a single component of the full complex (vitamin C and vitamin E are great examples of this) and convinced us that it was the same as eating an orange (vitamin C) or sunflower seeds (vitamin E). In reality it is not the same and these forms can rob your body of nutrients as it utilizes its reserves in an attempt to turn the counterfeits into something it can use. Additionally the synthetic versions of vitamins are simply toxic to your body. Remember the Cavemen? (If he didn't consume synthetic nutrients, neither should you.)

By the way this is another reason to avoid processed foods - they are often fortified with synthetic nutrients.

**As a side note, if you are not menstruating then you should get a Multi-vitamin formulation that does not have iron in it.

Companies that I trust: Garden of Life (Vitamin Code – Raw), New Chapter, Mega Food, AOR (though be picky as not all products will be Foodform/Whole complex), Dr. Mercola (www.mercola.com), Suzy Cohen (www.suzy-cohen.com)

Vitamin D3: Though it's called a vitamin it is actually a hormone. And a hormone is a fancy name for something that plugs into different places in your body and tells it how to behave. Vitamin D has over 300 sites to plug into throughout your body! It's a really important nutrient (along with Vitamin A… and conveniently they're both in butter and cod liver oil).

Most people are deficient in vitamin D so it is something (along with a good multi) that I recommend to everyone, especially from September 21st to April 21st when we can't possibly make vitamin D from the sun (in North America). And isn't it interesting that the time of the year that we can't get vitamin D from the sun is the same time that we have "cold & flu season"? So you can imagine how important it is for keeping your immune system healthy. It will also help with your mood and it can modulate your immune system so that if it is over-stimulated and attacking things that it shouldn't be, vitamin D will settle it down.

And this is interesting… a case of extreme skin itching for 10 years that was 98% relieved just by taking vitamin D. Her blood levels initially showed that she was super-deficient in the nutrient. (*the Vitamin D Revolution* by Soram Khalsa, M.D.)

How much to take is very controversial. Dr. Mercola (www.mercola.com) recently wrote that the average size adult needs 8,000 IU's daily. We also know that people who carry more weight (especially around the mid-section) may need more than an average sized person because the extra fat cells will steal the nutrient for themselves. If you're supplementing with a good source of D3 then toxicity is generally not a concern unless you've taken 25,000 IU's daily for 3 weeks. Likely 8,000 to 12,000 IU's will be a good daily dose for many adults, but it is highly recommended to have your doctor monitor your vitamin D levels so that you have an idea how much to take in order to keep it in a healthy range (see below).

50 ng/ml (and under) is considered deficient

50-70 ng/ml is considered optimal (higher for treating chronic diseases)

100 ng/ml is considered excessive and potentially toxic

The sun is the ideal source of vitamin D but is not always available or adequate (depending on the time of year, where you live, your age and skin colour) so the above guidelines will help you with a good D3 supplement. (Also, consider taking vitamin K2 with your D3. This is very new information so do your own research and decide for yourself. But the vitamin D is a must for LS healing.)

B – Complex: So many of us need to be taking a good B-complex or ideally, eating foods that are high in the B's. (Sadly because of soil depletion, busy schedules and the quantities needed, getting our needs met by food isn't always possible). Be certain it is the full complex, not a single B like B12 or B6 (and Suzy Cohen teaches to be certain the B12 is always Methyl, NOT Cyanocobalamin) though if you need extra, you can take a single B along *with* your B-complex. Even though your multi will have some B's in it, likely it won't be enough because our modern super-woman lifestyles really deplete the B's from us. Additionally if you've been using topical steroid ointment (and/or other medications like the Birth Control Pill), you're likely deficient in the B vitamins. Tip: if you suffer from anxiety - specifically a feeling of impending doom - and are chronically fatigued, then B's are likely part of your solution. (Don't be concerned if your urine becomes a bright yellow while taking B's!)

Vitamin C: In her book (*The Forbidden Truth about Vitamins What You Don't Know Will Hurt You*) Aleks reminded me that tissues get their strength and integrity from vitamin C. At the time, I only took extra C if I was feeling under the weather because I was on a multi. But (holy cow!) skin is a tissue and mine had lost its strength and integrity, at least in my greater vaginal area. When you think about it, this makes sense because vitamin C is an amazing antioxidant. What is an antioxidant? Think of your car left out in the elements year after year with no rust protection. Rust is oxidation and you don't want that happening in your body. But as I thought more and more of the connection between vitamin C deficiency and LS, I realized that the external symptoms did kind of resemble "rust".

What I had failed to consider (in my multi-vitamin-is-enough magical thinking) was that our food simply doesn't have the vitamin C in it that it used to and that the amount in my multi wasn't enough. Multi's aren't meant to cure deficiencies, only help to prevent them in the first place. But how did

I become deficient in vitamin C? This is a complex topic and there are a number of answers but here are a few of the key reasons… 1. I'm a human; humans are one of the only animals that don't make their own (essential nutrient) vitamin C. 2. I was under a lot of stress. And it turns out that along with cortisol and adrenaline, when you're under stress the Adrenal glands will also secrete precious vitamin C! 3. I wasn't taking in enough through foods or supplementation. 4. I had Hypothyroidism and the thyroid requires a great deal of vitamin C to be healthy. Can you see (or "C"!) yourself in this picture?

It is vitally important that you use the full complex of vitamin C not just the synthetic version called ascorbic acid. The companies I mentioned earlier have great vitamin C supplements. (Don't be afraid to take a higher dose especially if you have other vitamin C deficiency symptoms like spongy, bleeding gums, easy bruising, scaly/dry/brownish skin, and/or you "catch" everything that goes around.)

The list of vitamin supplements could go on and on but if you make all of the recommended changes in this book (especially with eating) plus take a multi (or you could do a multi one day and a good Whole Food Greens powder the next), you'll be taking in a lot more nutrients than you were when you first cracked the cover! So start with this basic list, and then see if you need to add others.

Essential Fatty Acids: EFA's for short. Just like vitamin C, this is an essential nutrient and your body does not make its own so you must take it in. You'd be amazed at all of the things that these essential fats do for your body (like take care of your heart and lower your inflammation!) but they are especially important for healthy <u>skin</u>, hair and nails. As I mentioned earlier, I learned from Suzy Cohen that to treat an eczema-like condition a 2-pronged approach with Fish oil AND Evening Primrose oil is really helpful. It moisturizes and lubricates from the inside out, plus it helps calm inflammation. Suzy recommends a 4 to 1 ratio so if you're taking 2,000mg's of Fish oil, to take 500mg's of Evening Primrose Oil (you can alternate the Evening Primrose

with Black currant or Borage oil if you like). But I haven't found a 500mg serving personally and so I take 1,000 mg's of each, 2 times daily and it works really well for me. Because my diet is so healthy, and full of other sources of EFA's, specifically Omega 3's, I am not concerned about the kind of Omega 6's found in Evening Primrose Oil. However, if you haven't committed to the dietary changes in the previous chapter, and still consume large amounts of processed foods and restaurant food, then you are getting too many inflammatory Omega 6's in your diet and it will hinder your progress in healing LS, as well as set you up for a myriad of other health problems down the road.

Astaxanthin: Even if you can't pronounce it, take it anyway because you'll love how it makes you look! Believed to be the most powerful antioxidant nature has to offer (remember you learned about oxidation when you read about vitamin C), it has a special affinity for your skin. And research shows that it makes people look younger in addition to making them healthier because it affects every cell in the body. The typical dose is 8mg's per day (taken in two 4mg doses) and you can expect to see results in 2 to 4 weeks. However the benefits to your inflamed LS skin will likely be noted much sooner. As with all recommended supplements, make certain you find natural Astaxanthin, not synthetic and then you'll never have to concern yourself with toxicity.

R-Lipoic Acid: You may have heard of *Alpha* Lipoic Acid and it will do if you need to save a bit of money but R-Lipoic is much easier for your body to use, so you'll get more benefit from it. We've talked so much about inflammation; here's a natural and safe "anti-inflammatory"! Suzy Cohen recommends R-lipoic acid along with Curcumin (coming up next) for treating diabetic neuropathy. That condition is one of THE most painful conditions known, so I figured if this combo could help the nerves feel better in that situation, they could help the nerve endings for the skin of my GVA! **Note that your urine may smell like asparagus when you use either R-lipoic or Alpha lipoic acid supplements.

Curcumin: This is the active ingredient from the spice turmeric. And feel free to use turmeric but it can be messy and you'll need a lot of it to get a therapeutic dose of Curcumin. Curcumin is an absolute blessing! It is an amazing

anti-inflammatory and it actually helps the cells in your body to heal. In fact, Curcumin can kill cancer stem cells (the "Mother" cells creating a tumor) but will strengthen the other cells of the body and make the immune system stronger (just the opposite of what chemo does). And here's something that might get your attention, in clinical trials Curcumin seems to have a particular affinity for inflammation around the waist, so it helps people (along with healthy eating as discussed) to lose weight, but especially around their bellies first!

The rest of my list has already been discussed in chapter 6 (the Candida one) but I'll remind you below. FYI I used Crude Candida Killers, Probiotics and the Barley Power for about 3 months only, at the beginning of this intensive healing process. However fermented foods and most supplements in this chapter continue to be part of my healthy routine.

Fermented Foods and/or Probiotics: Be sure to read
chapter 6 (Is Candida part of your LS picture?) if you haven't done so already. These foods or supplements will re-populate good (and needed) bacteria in your gut, ergo the rest of your body so that your immune system will be strong and can function optimally again.

Examples of fermented foods are: sauerkraut; kimchi; organic kefir; organic, plain yogurt with active bacteria; pickles (without vinegar) and kambucha. Do not purchase anything that is not in the refrigerator as it will no longer have live, active bacteria.

Depending on your situation you may need to start with just a probiotic supplement because the foods cause you "die off" symptoms. For others, or as your healing progresses, you may choose to use a probiotic in addition to eating fermented foods. I love Renew Life's probiotics (renewlife.ca or .com) because this company really knows its stuff about your gut. That said, Dr. Mercola has one that is shelf stable, meaning it does not have to be refrigerated, and he really knows his stuff too!

Crude Candida Killers: You'll definitely want to employ some
herbal help to get the population of Candida back down to a manageable

level. Some well-known Candida destroyers include: Oregano oil; Olive leaf extract; Pau d'arco; Garlic; Neem; Black Walnut; Apple cider vinegar; Caprylic acid; Coconut oil and Garlic. If you go to a reputable health food store, they're sure to have some great formulations for Candida.

Barley Power by Green Supreme (www.greensupreme.net):
Barley greens are amazing for making your body inhospitable to Candida! I took about 20 daily (they aren't very big and I stretched them through the day) along with my other Candida measures, and I felt I no longer suffered with Candida symptoms at about week 3. As a side benefit, these have over 3,000 enzymes in them, so you can skip taking an additional digestive enzyme if you choose them. (You may be able to find other barley greens at your local health food store. However this is an excellent company and it offers the convenience of tablets.)

Supplements to Avoid for
Eczema-like Skin Conditions:
I've used the term "eczema-like" a few times now and that's because I am convinced that Lichen Sclerosis is a form of eczema… for lack of a better term. In my clinical and personal experience it is much more like eczema than psoriasis. And that's an important distinction according to Suzy Cohen, because (as she explains in Eczema, Itchin' For a Cure) psoriasis is an Auto-immune condition but eczema is not.

That may be a bit confusing because we have discussed the immune system attacking things that it shouldn't so many times in this book already, but in the case of an auto-immune condition, if you had eliminated all other potential triggers (by fixing your diet and avoiding things you are sensitive/allergic too, etc.) then the immune system would still be attacking the skin for some (likely genetic) reason. But the great news is this does not appear to be the case with LS!

Ms. Cohen does a bang-up job of explaining the science behind all of this (in lay-man's terms) so if you want to understand it, check out her book.

But the super-important point here is that if you're dealing with an ecze-ma-like skin condition then it makes sense to avoid things that will over stimulate a Th2 dominant immune system. (That's what you'll learn... ec-zema suffers are largely Th2 dominant and have an immune system whose "B" cells are attacking and creating antibodies.) But guess what? Certain super-immune boosting supplements will make this situation worse! This was the case for me. I was taking some of these supplements because they're so good for us (we're told). And they are, but it's kind of like the Blood Type eating – with eating and supplements it turns out, that one size does NOT fit all.

Avoid, or exercise extreme caution (these will stimulate your Th2 domi-nant immune system and potentially cause LS Symptoms):
Caffeine
EGCG (In Green Tea) – take note blood type A's and AB's!
Grape Seed Oil
Lycopene
Oils – Safflower, Soy, Canola, Corn & Sunflower (mostly oils to avoid anyway!)
Pine Bark Extract
Pycnogenol
Resveratrol
White Willow Bark

Recommended to soothe and modulate your immune system so that it behaves in your best interest:
Probiotics*   EFA's *
Vitamin D*   Colostrum
Vitamin A   Boswellia
Vitamin E   Curcumin*

Lucky for you, half of these are already in your treatment plan! (Noted with the *) Additionally vitamins A and E will be in your multi vitamin but you can certainly experiment with taking more E on its own, and maybe adding a Cod Liver Oil supplement to get the perfect form of vitamin A (bring down your vitamin D if you do this, so that you won't be taking too much of it).

To be clear, my advice here is… start with what we've already covered in this chapter, but if you're not responding as quickly as you'd like, then consider adding in something else from this second list, and seeing how you do.

CHAPTER 10

Nourishing your spirit to heal your body

ARE YOU CAUGHT up in the (false) belief that your life will be better once your Lichen Sclerosis is? I know I was! (Read on to discover the truth…)

While I've given you a plethora of guidelines to help you recover from Lichen Sclerosis, I want to stress that there is no food plan, no Homeopathic remedy and no supplement that will replace your most basic requirements for sunshine, fresh air, being among living things (like trees) and love.

"And the greatest of these is LOVE". Often we look outside of ourselves for love. In fact we (women especially) are really bad at giving ourselves love. But look at it this way… imagine that you have a three year old girl in your charge (you may be her mother, aunt, guardian; it doesn't matter). Now imagine that she is overweight and that she isn't as cute as some other little girls that you've seen. (And every time you look at her, you feel less-than because you think she is a reflection of you.) Finally you've had enough, so you tell her: *I do not like the way that you look and I don't like your body! I am not going to feed you very much, and certainly you'll get nothing that you love to eat, until you look the way that I want you to.*

I know *YOU* would never treat a child this way, and yet this is exactly how women in Western cultures treat their bodies. Often I have to point this out to my patients who want to lose weight, but ladies it applies to the LS pathology too. It becomes a vicious circle because the angrier you are and the more ashamed you are at your body for "doing this thing to you," the more it helps to create the very pathology that you're angry about.

This can be a tricky concept to get, but it is worth understanding. If you attempt to change something about yourself - anything at all - without Love you will not have lasting results. Why? Substitute the word *Love* for *Power* in that last sentence. Not knowing (ergo not cultivating) *Divine* Love for yourself cuts you off from your Power.

Somewhere after our physical birth, we lose the knowledge that we are magnificent creatures worthy of more Love than we could ever imagine! Indeed we *are* Love, yet forget that too. Then, just when our parents have to let go, to let us make our way in the world (when we need Love the most), is right when we decide to cut ourselves off from Love. Most people around the ages of seventeen thru twenty-seven or twenty-eight are not "in Love" but "in Ego." (And many of us get stuck there for a lot longer!) We get caught up in this "outer" world of form and illusion. And then we take on the belief that if we were just somehow different (prettier, thinner, smarter, bustier, richer, *LS symptom free*, etc.) things would be better. The problem here is that the underlying operating system is flawed. If you attempt to change something about yourself because you don't Love yourself (read: because you feel powerless/cut off from your Source), then even if it seems to work for a time, eventually the problem will recur or a new, similar one will take its place. This happens because the underlying reason for the problem (lack of Love/Power) was not resolved - only suppressed for a time with a new focus. That's just how it works. It's a spiritual law that plays out over and over in the physical world, until you get it.

So the truth is: Your LS will be better when your life is better (because you'll have found your Divine Love/Power).

To understand the concepts introduced in this chapter better, head to your favourite book store and check out such authors as: Greg Braden, Wayne Dyer, Louise Hay, Esther Hicks, Florence Scovel Shinn, Tosha Silver; Neale Donald Walsch; Marianne Williamson, and so many more...! See which ones "speak" to you.

Right about now I bet you're thinking... *"But she didn't sound like she had very much love going on when she wrote that hate letter to God!"* And you'd be right. I had reached my (metaphoric) moment on the cross where I believed I was completely cut off from LOVE. But it was only a belief. I was wrong. And it took months of working with that little monk before I realized how worthy I was of the love *he* offered... and if I was worth that kind of love, I must certainly be worthy of *my* love! You see my healing was not instantaneous. It unfolded every few weeks for well over a year. At the beginning, while I struggled with being worthy of this "miracle" I was suppressing my (lack-of-LOVE) symptoms with cortisone cream. There was still a lot of work for me to do! But as I continued the spiritual journey and followed so much of what I've shared in this book, my life became better – in ways I'd never dared to imagine! And that's when my symptoms were gone... *when my life got better my LS got better.*

So let me save you some time. Hey, I'd love it if each of you got a call from a monk who could help liberate all of your shame and anger so that you could finally reach the Love (Power) that was in you all along! But that isn't very likely to happen. Instead, you get me :O)

I have been in your shoes and I am (now) on the other side telling you that you are so worth this journey! And it begins with LOVE. Today commit to a new habit... when you're washing your face each morning, take a really good look in the mirror (with love not judgement... if judgement comes up just cancel it by thinking: "I see The Divine in you.") and ask that *Divine Being* what she would like today. As often as you can, give that to yourself... just as if you were that three year old girl who so deserves the Power of your Love. Starting now be that loving care-giver that you need; that you deserve, and watch your true self unfold – with healthy body in tow. *Namaste!*

Bonus: EFT script for LS suffering relief
(Special thanks to "The Tapping Solution" folks for the use of their Tapping Points Chart!!)

EFT STANDS FOR Emotional Freedom Technique or "Tapping". It is a fast and effective way to get relief from nearly anything, *right now*. In a nutshell, tapping on ancient meridian points while you are feeling emotions and even physical symptoms, helps to unfreeze your Autonomic Nervous System so that you can feel okay again. Simple right?!

For more information on tapping I encourage you to check out Nick Ortner's The Tapping Solution book(s) and documentary... (www.thetappingsolution.com)

Admittedly I am a newbie when it comes to tapping but I am sold!! In a few short weeks I feel like it's changed my life. In fact, it even helped me to get this book to you! But while I was finishing it, I was going through a challenging life event and I developed a really itchy rash on most of my body (but happily not on my genitals!). Eventually I did find the right Homeopathic remedies but one night the itching was pretty intense and I suddenly remembered the tapping course I was taking. I muddled though with the language and really focused on my feelings (fear), and no kidding, in about 6 minutes the itching had subsided from a 10 to a 2!

Nick (Ortner) suggests that you check in with yourself before you tap, so that you have a starting point to gauge from. Ask yourself: on a scale of 1 to 10 (1 being hardly noticeable and 10 being the worst ever) how bad is the itching and/or pain right now? When you have that number you can write it down, and then ask yourself if there is an emotion or a few emotions that go along with (or are underneath) the itching and/or pain. When you have that answer you're ready to tap.

The tapping points (in order)

1   Karate Chop Point (the point on your dominant hand if you were going to chop through a piece of wood)
2   Inner eye brows
3   Outer corner of eyes
4   Under the eyes
5   Under the nose
6   Chin
7   Collar bone (where those two bones kind of meet)
8   Under the arms (on your rib cage)
9   Top of the head

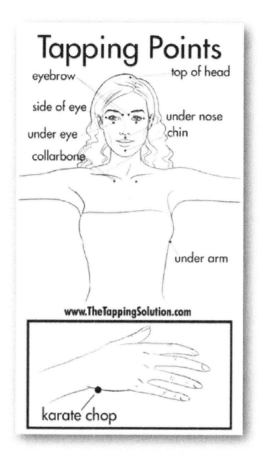

Tapping Script for Itching/Pain:

(You may want to do it a few times if you have both itching and pain or you can combine them)

Here we go (use both hands where applicable)... begin by using your least dominant hand to tap on the karate chop point of your dominant hand and say the following "Set Up" statement:

Karate Chop: Even though I have this horrific itching that is all consuming and ruining my life, I deeply and completely accept myself (say this 3 times)

Now tap on the points as you go through the script…

Eyebrow: This itching

Side of eye: This itching of my genitals

Under eye: I am ashamed to say that and think it even, but it is taking so much of my energy

Under nose: Attempting not to scratch takes so much of my attention

Chin: Scratching is all I think about and the doctors say there is no cure for this condition; this itching

Collarbone: If there's no cure, I'm going to have this itching all of my life and I feel scared and overwhelmed

Under arms: I am so unbelievably itchy and the more I think about it the more frightened I become

Top of head: This horrible itching! What if it never goes away?

Now go through this a few times (from Eyebrow point) until you feel like it is beginning to settle or you feel calmer.

Then proceed...

Eyebrow: Hmm, it seems like the itching isn't so bad now

Side of eye: Is this possible? Yes, I am feeling better

Under eye: Even though the doctors said there's no cure, I am feeling better

Under nose: Wow, the itching is so much better and now I don't feel overwhelmed and afraid

Chin: Maybe I don't have to suffer with this for the rest of my life, and I have tapping to help me whenever I need it

Collarbone: I am really feeling better; the itching is so much better and I am not afraid anymore

Under arms: I can't believe how much better I feel; even my shame about this condition has lessened

Top of head: This is so simple and it works; I feel so much better

*Feel free to repeat this section as many times as you'd like and then...

Take a deep breath in through your nose... and out through your mouth.

Now check in with yourself to see where your number is at. You may want to repeat the process until you get it to a 2 or lower, but you can also stop for now, if you're satisfied with how much better you feel. *Do use tapping as often as you need for quick symptom relief!

Tapping may seem a bit cumbersome or awkward at first but don't worry, you'll get it, and keep in mind that you don't have to be perfect at it! But just in case you're struggling, I have two options for you...

1. Take a tip from Nick and simply have a conversation with your best friend. You can be on the phone (with a hands-free device) telling her all about your LS and how you're now on this journey to heal it, and just do the tapping while you're talking. (Hint, this works with praying too!)
2. Head to my website (www.quick-health.ca) and tap along (and repeat after me) to an extended audio version of this script.

Printed in Great Britain
by Amazon

37757127R00071